Intermittent Fasting For Women

The 14-Days Pyramid-Fasting To A Slimmer You.

The Essential Step-by-Step Guide For Serious Fat Reduction, Body Self-Cleansing With Autophagy And Healthy Lifestyle.

By Linda Samson

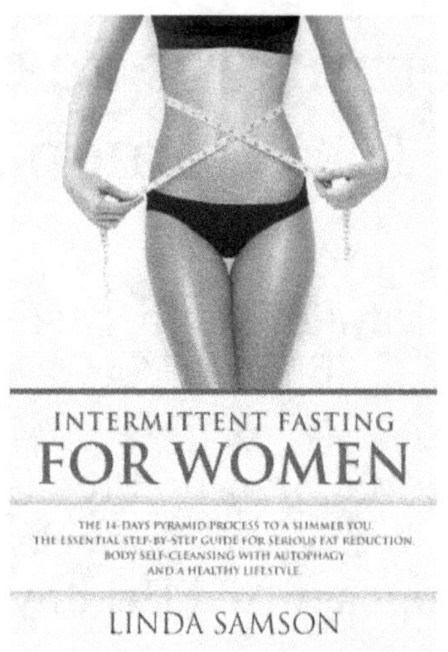
INTERMITTENT FASTING
FOR WOMEN
THE 14-DAYS PYRAMID-PROCESS TO A SLIMMER YOU.
THE ESSENTIAL STEP-BY-STEP GUIDE FOR SERIOUS FAT REDUCTION.
BODY SELF-CLEANSING WITH AUTOPHAGY
AND A HEALTHY LIFESTYLE.
LINDA SAMSON

Table of Contents

Introduction

This book is designed to introduce you to the facts about Intermittent Fasting (IF) and why it's the perfect diet plan for women. Find out why women struggle so much to lose extra pounds and how IF can cut through the red tape, giving you optimal, lasting results. You will know exactly what needs to be done to start your customized IF plan by the time you finish this book.

The health benefits go way beyond losing stubborn body fat. It holds the keys to improving brain function, immune system response, lowers blood sugar, reduced inflammation, detoxification of the entire body, and promotion of your healing capabilities. The continued practice of IF can provide a lifetime of benefits and even promote a longer lifespan.

You have the opportunity to create your own customized IF plan with the included instructional sections that explain what to do and why. Everything is explained easily and in a way that makes sense. You will fully understand everything there is to know about IF, autophagy, and how it all benefits women today and will continue to be an important solution for lagging metabolism.

You will learn what foods are good and which ones are to be avoided in order to assist in your body's ability to turn fat into energy. You'll begin melting away pounds of fat from your first fast. Be prepared to open new avenues of opportunity for improving your health and speeding your weight loss goals along.

IF is a weight loss and healthy dieting routine that works if you are a woman that is serious about losing unwanted pounds, as well as completely rejuvenate every cell in your body. Take as much time as you need to choose your perfect plan and customize it to meet your specific goals. Get ready to look and feel like a brand-new woman!

Chapter 1: Intermittent Fasting (IF) – The Women's Diet

The search for a diet that provides increased energy, leaner muscles, and incredible fat burning results has been ongoing for decades. Scientific studies increasingly point towards the things you DON'T eat being more influential than what you DO eat. More specifically, the times you eat compared to fasting periods help determine the final outcome. Intermittent fasting offers the most flexibility in menu, eating times, and nearly effortless weight-loss.

What is Intermittent Fasting?

Most people practice some level of intermittent fasting, whether they realize it or not. If you eat dinner at 6 pm, put little more in your system beyond water for the night and eat breakfast at 8 am the next morning, you have fasted for 14-hours. It is one reason that intermittent fasting is an easier diet for many to follow. You can sleep much of the time away, although longer fasting times will require some effort.

Intermittent fasting splits your time into two categories. Any of the hours you are able to eat are called the **Fed State**. The hours designated to be without calories are called the **Fast State**. It's a way to sensibly divide calorie intake through hours, rather than extensive calorie counting at all times of the day or night. You know that during fast hours, you are limited to drinking items that are calorie-free, such as water or unsweetened tea and coffee.

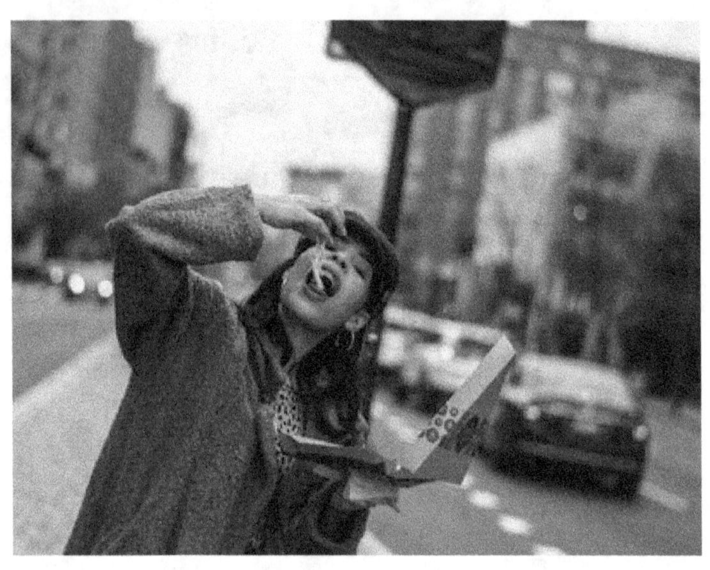

Self-Control and Healthy Eating Habits

Two skills that will carry you far with IF is strong self-control and healthy eating habits. You need to be able to stick out the times of fasting without breaking it unless you have no other options. Self-control is also required when you hit the feeding hours following the fast. The urge to eat too much to satiate hunger can lead to stomach aches or gaining weight. Developing healthy eating habits will keep you from overeating during your designated meal hours.

It's a natural way to restrict calories without being consumed with finding the specific foods needed to fit your dieting plans. You can eat what you want without fearing that you're setting yourself up for failure. IF is about sensibly cutting down on calories rather than trying to make up for all you missed out on during the fast.

The concept of the IF diet is a great one for women as long as all precautions are taken to do the diet correctly. Not following the dietary regimen can cause imbalances of hormones and other problems that are not specific to one gender, but affect women in a harsher measure. Not many studies have been conducted on humans, but have been primarily done with rats. Much of the problems associated with IF have been documented by those experiencing difficulties. It's helped develop a clearer picture of IF in action.

This book will give you all the information you need to make a better decision as to whether IF is the right diet plan for you. The ability to customize a fasting routine that works best for your needs gives you greater odds of successfully sticking with the plan. IF, used over time, can be an incredibly effective way to generate more energy out of the foods you eat.

IF and the Female Body

Everything about the female body and its internal functions is somewhat different from men. Both men and women have kidneys, heart, liver, eyes, and hair, but the process of female digestion, pain recognition, and nutrient collection is not the same as it is for men. IF can help with everything from immune system boost to greater metabolic efficiency.

Insulin Sensitivity and Women

Insulin sensitivity can be heightened in women. Females are much more sensitive to the slightest fluctuations in blood sugar. When IF is done correctly, you can expect that your blood sugar levels and insulin sensitivity will be at levels that are tolerable. Not paying attention to these issues and running headlong into too rigorous a fast can lead to health problems.

The key for successful IF experiences in women is taking time to build up to each stage and finding one your body fits comfortably. There is no one-plan-fits-all with fasting. There's not even a single plan for women and another for men. Each person has such an individual constitution that it must be created as you go to fit personal needs and body responses.

Starvation Response in Women

One area that differs between men and women using the IF diet method is the starvation response. Whether a woman is pregnant or not, fasting can sometimes trigger a strong starvation response. The body will begin socking away every calorie for sustaining through a perceived food drought. It can render the IF experience useless. You'll gain weight no matter what you do.

Taking the process reasonably slow and allowing your body to adjust at each stage is what makes the difference. The female body can get used to the IF routine and adjust in safe and comfortable ways. You will find that the two-week pyramid system introduced in this book provides the perfect foundation for each step in the plan. You can see real results at every level.

Why IF is the Perfect Diet Plan for Women

The fact that a woman's body is sensitive to the subtle changes in blood sugar is not a disadvantage when you can more immediately tell if there is a problem. It can be used to your advantage. Immediate adjustments can be made to your plan that puts you back on the right track. It allows you to end a fast right away to avoid a serious health problem. The sensitive nature of the female biological makeup is not a bad thing.

The uncomplicated nature of IF is the biggest reason that it is possibly the best diet plan for a woman to follow. Much of the fasting can be done during sleep hours. It limits the feeling of food restriction. Nothing is more appealing than a diet that doesn't feel like deprivation and food torture. You are allowed to eat a wide selection of good foods during your designated eating periods. No part of creating and following through with the IF plan is difficult to understand or follow.

Autophagy

The remarkable process called autophagy is something that can team up with your IF efforts and provide faster results than you might expect. It can boost metabolism and provide a deep cleansing action to improve the way your body functions. It goes well beyond anything a chemical detox product could do. One great thing is you have no idea it is happening. It is automatic, much like breathing or your heartbeat.

What is Autophagy?

Autophagy is a process in the body that happens at the cellular level that naturally cleans up the cells, spaces between the cells, and helps determine what cells are used to create the energy your body needs. You have designated cells that manage the autophagy process. These cells can be stimulated or triggered to boost or extend their natural behaviors.

One of the best triggers for autophagy is fasting, in any form. There is no form of IF plan that is any better at triggering than another. In other words, you have just as much opportunity to benefit from autophagy by short fasts as you would by long fasts. The maximum window of autophagy benefit is 2-days. It peaks at 12 hours and drops off after 48 hours. Choosing a fast of 14-24 hours will give your body plenty of time to benefit from autophagy.

How IF Benefits Autophagy

The most obvious initial way that IF benefits the autophagy process is by triggering. Autophagy is going on in the background, but not at the super level that triggering provides. Increasing the activity of autophagy means a complete detox that purges old cells, cellular parts, and removal of viruses, bacteria, or other pathogenic matter. You are actually helping your immune system by fasting.

Allowing the cells of your body to thrive in a healthier environment, free of harmful materials and cellular garbage means that every organ and structure in your system will operate more efficiently. Less difficulty in gaining energy and releasing wastes will keep cells from prematurely aging and dying.

The cells responsible for autophagy are able to selectively determine which cells to eat up for energy. The immediate reduction in carbs and sugars with the fasting of IF helps steer the autophagy cells to burn stored fats. It directly impacts your fat burning capabilities. The weight loss experienced is steady and direct. The muscles you have will be made leaner without any extra effort.

Are there bad side effects to autophagy?

The natural use and encouragement of the autophagy process are relatively harmless, but as with anything, you need to make sure that your activity level is monitored when at high-level or peak autophagy. If you are going slow enough, the cells of the body can carefully decide which cells to sensibly eat for energy. Going too speedily into a deep fast will trigger the autophagy to a point that you should not do much in the way of physical exertion. Your body will begin breaking down muscular tissue as if you were literally starving in a desert. Easy-does-it is the key.

A few benefits of autophagy you can expect are:

- Deep detox of the body
- Increased weight loss
- Fewer illnesses like colds and flu

- Increased clarity of thought
- Youthful, energetic feeling
- Diminishing of hunger pangs during the fasting state

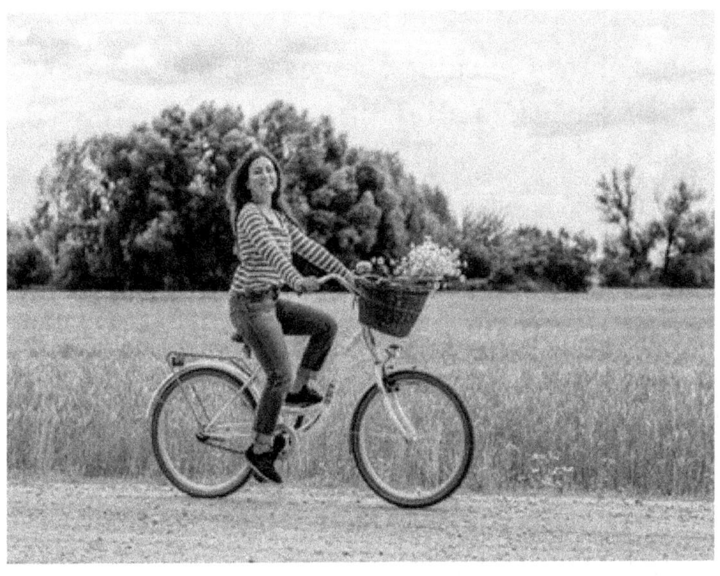

Protein Cycling

The average woman is said to consume at least 70 grams of protein each day. It's 1.5 times more than the amount needed by the body. The excess will be stored up in the body as fat. It works against your efforts to lose weight with IF. You must do protein cycling to get the maximum benefits of autophagy and intermittent fasting.

Glucagon and Insulin

One of the delicate balances you have to look at closely when attempting to lose weight with IF is the levels of glucagon and insulin. The periods of fasting that are without food will increase the levels of glycogen in your system. Periods of eating are marked by an immediate increase in insulin. The balance will shift from one to the other, depending on which part you are in.

The fasting part of IF that increases glycogen triggers the start of autophagy. The cells in charge of autophagy are desperately looking for anything to use in place of the protein and carbs they are used to accessing through meals and snacking. Exiting the fast and entering the fed state reduces the autophagy to normal maintenance levels. Maximizing the autophagy action is where weight loss happens in more noticeable levels.

The Benefits of Protein Deprivation

Depriving the body of protein is another way to trigger autophagy. The cells responsible will seek out every area to gather protein, when available, to convert to energy. Without it, the results are burning fat. It's a desirable outcome for anyone using food intake controls as a way to remove stubborn fat deposits anywhere on the body.

It's not practical to think that you can totally deprive your body of protein to lose a ton of weight. It can be unhealthy and unwise. Protein deprivation has to be used on a rotational basis, rather than over consecutive days of the week. Otherwise, your body will begin to break down existing muscle protein in the false belief you are actually starving.

Low and High Cycles

Combining the ability to increase autophagy with fasting and protein deprivation can intensify the benefits. You can carefully do this as long as you are mindful of having a few days of a full protein-normal diet. You do this by creating a low cycle day that includes fasting and finishing with a low-protein fed state. The next day, you will enjoy a 24-hour non-fast day with a normal diet. Your schedule would look something like this:

Monday: 16-hour fast (partially through the previous night), remaining 8-hours lite protein diet.

Tuesday: Normal diet.

Wednesday: 16-hour fast (partially through the previous night), remaining 8-hours lite protein diet.

Thursday: Normal diet.

Friday: 16-hour fast (partially through the previous night), remaining 8-hours lite protein diet.

Saturday: Normal diet.

Sunday: 16-hour fast (partially through the previous night), remaining 8-hours lite protein diet.

Alternating days gives you the opportunity to utilize the maximum fat burning assistance of autophagy and still remain intaking the nutrients your body needs to stay healthy. It's a beautiful balance that gives you real results in dropping inches from your waistline fast.

IF and Hormones

The long-running myth that IF can drastically affect the hormones of a woman is only true if you completely disregard your overall health and have a pre-existing condition that easily leads to hormonal troubles. When done properly, most women report experiencing more stable moods, less periods of emotional-based eating, and steady weight loss. Although very few studies exist for humans, the ones available point towards the need to start gentle, stay steady, and ease off when or if you don't feel right. Stress added on top of the stress that IF adds to the body is often responsible for throwing hormones out of whack.

The Stress of Feeling Hungry

Jumping up in stages too quickly with your IF plan can leave you feeling food-deprived and stressed. Make sure you give yourself the full two-weeks to adjust to the level you are on before getting more intense. Your body will already feel stress from the switch to burning fat due to less carbs and proteins.

Feel free to add a cup of broth to your fast period or some unsweetened coconut fat to your cup of tea if you are feeling stressed about hunger pains. It does technically break the fast, but continue as if nothing happened. Anything to break the stress can be more beneficial than trying to struggle through.

Skipping the Cortisol Stressor

The natural response to the body wanting and needing food is a drop of blood sugar levels. Your body will begin to flood hormones that are specific to telling you to eat. If this goes ignored, the body steps things up a notch. It sends cortisol out to make your feelings of hunger more intense. It adds a tremendous amount of stress to the body.

The easiest way to avoid the stress of cortisol is to make sure you are eating plenty of dense, calorie-enriched foods. Take your time to eat well and plenty during the fed state. Eat foods with high amounts of good fats like nuts and grass-fed meats. You'll nearly eliminate the hunger pains and the fasting state will be more comfortable.

Thyroid and Hormone Imbalance

You need to monitor the symptoms you feel if you have an existing thyroid problem that throws your hormone levels off-balance. Extreme hormone imbalances can impact your internal temperature controls, mood, appetite, and can lead to menopause starting earlier than it should. Periods can completely disappear. Have your hormone levels checked if you begin having problems that seem associated with hormones. A thyroid that is over or under operating causes tremendous imbalances in the levels of hormones in the female body.

Know When to Quit

Pay attention to any signals your body is giving. If you are feeling bad for any reason, stop the fast. It is better to break one day of fasting than end up with health problems. It won't be hard to get back on track. Distraction is another thing that causes you to lose focus and trip. Be kind to yourself and try again. Missing one day of fast will not kill the whole process.

Pros and Cons of the IF Lifestyle

As with any dietary changes that are new, you will find a fair share of positives and negatives. The IF plan is one that takes a little pre-planning and fortitude to stick with the fast. Your baseline nutrition is critical to continuing with a measure of success. Intermittent fasting is a diet method that can easily become a lifestyle once you settle on the right type and level that comfortably fits your needs and schedule. Let's look at some of the noted pros and cons of IF.

Pros of the IF Lifestyle

IF is affordable

The intermittent fasting diet requires no special foods beyond healthy items you'd want to eat anyway. You might have to switch out the types of meat you buy for grass-fed varieties and eat less carbs, but it's not an expensive change to make. You do not have to take a bunch of supplements and additives that are costly and budget-killing.

IF is flexible

You'll find out how flexible it is in the upcoming chapter about the different types of IF. It allows you to choose a program that works with your schedule and ability to stick with the routine.

IF works whether or not you exercise

The increase of fat burning by autophagy in the fasting period means exercise is not required to begin losing weight. Regular exercise is a good thing to maintain a healthy heart but IF produces results even if you don't spend hours each day at the gym.

No food deprivation during the fed state

You can eat what you want during the fed state, which means you should never feel food deprived during those hours. Filling up adequately on food will ensure you feel less hunger pangs during the fast. The use of high-density foods gives the ultimate sensation of being full and having your hunger satisfied.

Consistent weight loss

The IF routine, when followed faithfully and correctly, will provide a slower and more consistent weight loss than many other types of diet. It's guaranteed to be permanent weight loss as long as you follow through with healthy eating activities. You will see inches of built-up fat melt away over a reasonable amount of time.

Supercharge fat burning

Intermittent fasting gives you the opportunity to use fat adapting and autophagy to increase the level of fat burning to incredible levels. You will lose weight in a steady way and feel confident that it's unwanted fat, rather than muscle tissue or water.

Cons of the IF Lifestyle

Weight loss slowing

You can reach a peak in IF where the weight loss will begin to level off and slow down. It's largely due to the eating done during the fed state. The more calories you pack in, the more the insulin will carry over to your fasting state. It places limits on the amount of fat burning done. You can keep this from happening by balancing the calories and making sure you only eat what is necessary to keep up your nutrition levels.

Inconvenient

IF isn't an impossibly difficult diet program to follow, but it has its moments of inconvenience. Being invited to dinner, luncheons, barbecues, and other eating-related gatherings can make you feel uncomfortable. Everyone that's present might wonder why you're only drinking black coffee or water. You have to be prepared to skip these events or answer questions.

Not universal

The IF plan is not one everyone can handle. You should check with your doctor and make sure that any type of fasting diet is possible. Certain medications and medical conditions make it impossible.

Controversial

Not everyone agrees with IF or a fasting diet. Some people consider it hipster or weird.

Some can't believe anyone would think of skipping the all-important breakfast meal. You need to understand from the outset that some people close to you will view it negatively

Complete commitment

Successful results with IF require a complete commitment to the fasting portions, which can be difficult at times. It's one of the most common listed difficulties with this diet plan. Much like anything, you'll only get out of it what you're willing to put in as far as effort and focus.

Chapter 2: IF Basics

Learning how to succeed with IF requires taking a closer look at what it is and how it works. This chapter will focus on why IF is the diet plan to choose, how to use IF, and a few things to reasonably expect as you progress.

Why Fasting?

Fasting has been practiced for thousands of years. It is historically known as a popular activity in a variety of religious communities in the past and present. Fasting briefly is a requirement before surgeries and other medical procedures. Fasting out of choice has not always been the norm. Many civilizations ran into problems that left the populace without adequate amounts of food. Forced fasts are what have adapted the body to function well for periods of time without outside food sources.

Increase Longevity, Reduce Disease, and Maintain Neuroplasticity

Consistently loading the body with calories is proven to make you live a shorter life, prone to neurodegenerative conditions like Alzheimer's and Parkinson's disease. It's impractical to continually deprive yourself of meals. Starvation methods with the goal of living longer can make your life miserable. Some level of IF is shown to benefit you by reducing the problems associated with aging and disease.

If your goal is to make your elderly years more pleasant and live a long time, you can begin a limited schedule of fasting that is not difficult or too food-restrictive. You can try the occasional meal skip or the 16:8, which allows you 8 hours each day to eat. You don't have to put yourself through hours and hours or days of fasting.

Burn Fat and Increase Metabolism

Burning fat and increasing metabolism leads to dramatic, permanent weight loss over time. Simply cutting back on calories can backfire and cause you to begin gaining weight. Your body can become concerned that you have entered a starvation period and will begin storing away everything possible as fat. IF is a way to train your body to burn the stored fat comfortably, causing you to benefit from weight loss.

Start with an easy twice a week fast and gradually work up to more intense routines, such as the Warrior diet or skip-eat-skip. Your metabolism will increase as you progress in stages.

Build and Create Lean Muscles

A goal of building muscle or getting your current muscles in a leaner condition will require a mix of the right exercise routines and IF. You'll want to gradually increase in the intensity of IF routines. The alternate day fasting and the16:8 work well as long as you make sure you are eating well within two or three hours of your workouts.

Make sure you add enough protein to your diet so that your body has the materials necessary to build new muscle tissue. You also need to add more carbohydrates than standard to have the energy levels required for working out.

Complete and Deep Detox

Taking advantage of increased autophagy activity to clean out your body of toxins and old cellular material is a major benefit of IF. It's an easy way to naturally keep every cell in your body in a more youthful, invigorated condition. All of this can be gained without the use of chemicals and tinctures, with a deeper detox result.

Detox and cleansing goals can be reached easily by starting with a simple 5:2 plan, which has you fasting two designated days of the week. You can then move on to a more aggressive alternating fast if you want to maintain the cleansed state.

Increase Strength and Power

Increasing your energy, strength, and literal power in your body is a careful balance of cleansing the cells for better performance and increasing metabolism. The faster you burn fat as energy, the more energy you'll have at your access.

The Warrior diet is a great IF plan that lets you pack in calories to the last 4 hours of your day. You can also try the 16:8, which is more flexible in allowing you to eat for 8 hours in the day. Both will increase the metabolic rate in the body and elevate your natural energy levels.

When to Fast

Higher levels of success and results can happen by carefully planning when you fast. Try and pick times that cause the least amount of stress and intrusion on your life. The calmer and easier it seems, the more likely it is you'll stick with the fasting.

Time of the Day

The time of the day that you commit to the fasting portion of IF can make a huge difference in your successful completion. If you are nervous about how bad the hunger pangs might be, try doing a majority of the hours of fast during the night. On a 12:12 plan with 12 hours of fast and 12 hours of eating window, do 8 hours of your fast as you sleep. If you begin your fast at a 9 pm window the night before, you can eat breakfast at 9 am and have a last meal for the next day complete by 9 pm.

If you are doing the 16:8 plan, start at 9 pm the night before and you'll be able to eat a meal at 1 pm the next day. You'll finish your last meal at 9 pm that night. A 24 hour fast starts at your designated 9 pm and ends the next day at 9 pm.

Days of the Week

Plans with built-in eating windows like the 12:12 or 16:8 can be followed the same way each day of the week for your fasting period.

You can begin slower by limiting the days to 3 or 4 for your first stage and gradually move towards every day.

Full fast days will be alternated or chosen days of the week. Try and pick your least stressful days of the week for full fasting. The stress of not eating calories and placing it on top of a hectic work or personal day can prove trying. Design a plan that allows you to succeed.

Why You Should Alternate Days of Full Fasting and Regular Diet

You can customize an IF plan to include full, 24-hour days of fasting. You can turn the 5:2 into a 4:3 and have 3 full 24-hour fasting days within the week and 4 regular diet days. The important thing when doing this is to make sure there is at least one day of regular diet between each 24-hour fast. It will help keep the glycogen and insulin balance necessary to keep stress at a minimum.

The stress of having glycogen and insulin at levels that are too high and low can send a woman into hormonal imbalance and cause blood sugar issues. An alternating day total fast will help you lose pounds faster but it must be done with care and thoughts of alleviating systemic stress.

What and How Much to Eat

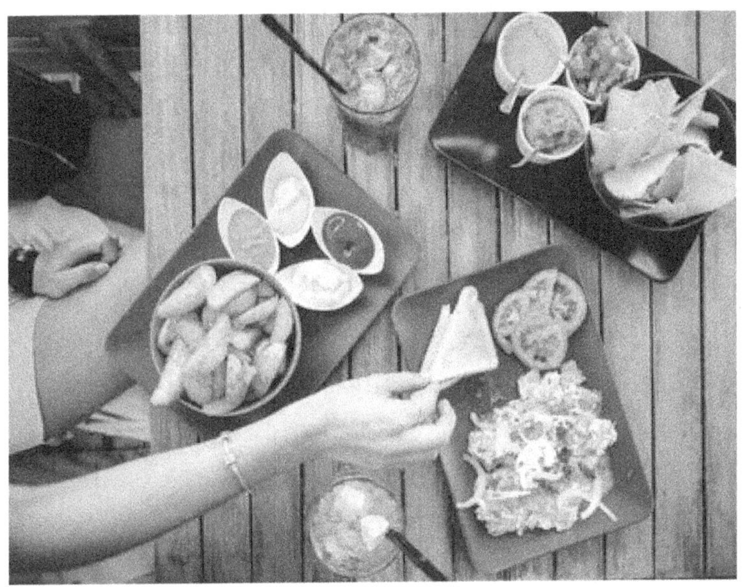

The foods and amounts you eat will be as important as the IF planned fasting window. It does no good to starve yourself for a whole day and then eat until you drop the next day. For one, you wouldn't feel good after that activity and second, you'll actually end up gaining weight. Sensible eating patterns and healthy foods are the best choices to make for meals and snacks.

The 65-30-5 Nutrition Intake Guide

When practicing the IF plan, you have to restrict carbohydrates more than fat or protein. For a normal IF diet, try and make the fat content 65 percent of your daily intake, 30 percent protein, and 5 percent carbs.

You need to change this up a little bit if you are doing heavy workouts or plan on being highly physically active. Change the amounts to 30 percent fats, 40 percent protein, and 30 percent carbs for the meal right before a period of intense physical activity.

Good Foods to Eat for IF

Fish
Fish is not only a good source of protein but it's also considered to be loaded with high levels of healthy fat. You should gather at least 40 percent of your weekly protein from fish.

Avocados
Avocado is a fruit that contains high levels of calories but it also helps keep your stomach full. It can aid in waiting out those long periods between meals.

Nuts
Nuts are a food that is teaming with healthy fats. It gives your body the materials needed to get used to burning fats for energy.

Eggs
Eggs are nearly the perfect protein. Each egg contains 6 grams of protein. It's an easy food to fix and can satisfy hunger quickly.

Beans or Legumes
Lentils, black beans, or chickpeas are all great sources of carbs that are light in calories. It also adds fiber to your diet that makes you feel fuller faster.

Fiber-Rich Vegetables
Cauliflower, broccoli, and Brussel's sprouts are all high fiber, high-density foods that help prevent constipation. It's important if you are

just beginning your IF journey. Dense, fibrous foods will also help you feel fuller, longer.

Portions and Meal Frequency

The portions you eat should be no more than you would, had you never fasted. The urge to load up your plate and binge eat must be curtailed for IF to work. You should not try and fit more than one meal and one snack into each 4-hour eating window.

Intermittent Fasting and the Keto Diet: An Ideal Pairing

No matter what IF plan you choose, you have to eat. The diet you choose to follow while on IF can hinder or help you in your progress. The keto diet is one that can not only help your weight loss and other health-related goals, but it can make the IF process more comfortable.

What is the Keto Diet?

The keto diet is one that drastically reduces carbs and sugars and forces the body into a state of ketosis, which is less dependence on glucose and insulin for energy. Your body becomes adapted to burning fat for fuel. Your body will not have to struggle in switching from having blood sugar elevated in the fed state and dropping off sharply during the fast.

The focus on increased fats and foods that are more filling that comprises the keto diet make it a natural choice to anyone considering starting the IF plan. For best results, begin eating a ketogenic diet a couple of weeks before you start your first phase of IF. You'll appreciate the benefits and better results.

Increasing Your Chance for Success

Being able to avoid the extreme up and down feeling of a normal diet laden with carbs and sugars and the sudden switch to fasting will make your system feel more stable. Your fat burning potential will be accelerated by the benefits of combining fasting triggered autophagy and ketosis. You will reach your goal weight faster and with less effort. The hunger pangs will suddenly disappear. Overall, the keto diet and IF are the perfect combination.

A clean fast is one in which you take in zero calories from food or drinks during the fasting portion. A modified fast can allow drinks that have tiny amounts of calories during the fast state. What you are trying to avoid is an insulin response, but it might not be possible to go completely without calories if you begin to feel dizzy or completely fatigued.

The Importance of Hydration

Your body gathers hydration not only from the liquids you drink but the foods you eat also contain moisture. Entering a fasting plan like IF means you will be restricting liquids from one portion for specified periods of time. You should increase your hydration slightly during your fast state. By slightly, it's wise to increase your water consumption by one glass each day. Base it on your thirst, but never overdo things.

Water as a Main Source of Hydration

Water is going to be your main source of hydration during any IF plan. It makes sense since it's a zero-calorie drink that the body needs daily. The average woman should drink eight to nine glasses of water each day. Increase this by one glass for every day of fasting. Spread the water consumption throughout the day and don't use it purely as a way to fill an empty stomach. Your body needs a steady source of hydration. Always bring cool water to drink with you when going out to avoid the temptation of purchasing high-calorie drinks.

Coffee, Tea, and Non-Calorie Drinks

Does hydration always have to come in the form of plain water? Of course, you can choose from other things that have high-water content. You need them to be calorie-free. Some good alternatives are coffee, tea, and electrolyte water. Avoid the name-brand sports drinks that are packed with chemicals and sugars your body doesn't need during a fast.

If caffeine is bothersome, switch to herbal teas and decaffeinated varieties of standard tea and coffee. Remember not to include milk, creamer, and sugar as it adds calories. You can use a small splash of low-calorie almond milk if you have no choice, but it puts a crimp in your clean fasting. Minimize the amount to avoid an insulin rush.

Fruit Infused Water and Broth

Lack of flavor can be more stressful than you realize during hours of fasting. It's nice to get a drink of water but it leaves you missing flavor. Try adding fruit to the water to infuse it with the natural flavor. The actual juice transfer is minimal and it can reduce your cravings for something more disastrous to your fast.

Hunger pangs can also be a problem if you find that your fed state is including more carbs and sugars than it should. You can begin to feel real effects from dipping blood sugar levels. You can combat this and stay somewhat on track by drinking vegetable, chicken, or beef broth. It's low-calorie and can kick the cravings for food right away. It's the perfect additive if you are not looking to maintain a complete calorie-free fast.

Not Counting Every Calorie

IF plans do not require you to count every calorie, with the exception of the plans that offer a restricted calorie intake between fasts. It's completely freeing to not be enslaved to constant calorie counting. You can enjoy food during your windows without feeling an ounce of guilt.

More Flexibility to Naturally Fit Your Schedule

If you ever wanted an unsuccessful and cumbersome diet strategy, try putting one in place that you must completely design your life around. Rigid rules and stipulations rarely work. You'll end up frustrated and giving up when it gets tough. Rules do apply with the IF plans but they are flexible enough to allow you the ability to customize one that works perfectly. It's not the end of the world if you fall off the fast for a day. Restart the next day as if nothing had happened. It provides true motivation to keep going. Every bit of progress is not lost in the process.

You Can Eat Whatever You Want in Fed State

The list of foods you CAN eat is much larger than what you should avoid. Most of the foods deemed bad for ketosis and autophagy for weight loss are not very healthy to eat anyway. IF gives you a great roadmap to head towards better health and a healthy body weight. The nearly open choices available give you something to look forward to when ending your fast. You don't have to make a meal for your family and a complete separate meal for yourself. It saves time and money.

Eating Out is Easier

Eating a restricted and limited diet can make eating out at restaurants or at family gatherings nearly impossible. You don't want to trouble family and friends to make specialized dietary foods. Restaurants don't always have food available that's friendly towards your needs. IF lets you eat a fairly normal diet, which makes it easier to find something you can eat without feeling guilt or giving long-winded explanations.

It is easier if you set your IF plan to coincide with eating windows at prime eating hours. Your chances will be greater that you aren't in a fasting period and can take advantage of the freedom to eat.

Simpler Weight Loss Method

The IF plan you choose will be a simpler and less-complicated way to achieve your goals than any you've tried before. Taking your focus off food can make life generally simpler. Beyond documenting you're eating habits at the beginning, very little needs to be tracked and counted. The only exception is for those using a restricted calorie eating window. You'll have to note when you've reached your available calorie count.

Easy to Restart if You Make a Mistake

Dropping blood sugar levels, extreme feelings of hunger, or feeling ill are all good reasons to discontinue a fast. It's better to be safe and make sure everything is okay before moving ahead. You can follow through with your eating window and move on to the next fast if you're feeling better at that time. If not, wait until things seem right and try it again.

Chapter 3: IF for Women

The IF method of using fasting to lose weight and improve your health can be used by women in all walks of life and for many specific benefits. Setting the stage for success will give you the improvements you need health-wise and help you drop fat reserves at unbelievably fast rates. This chapter explores some of the benefits enjoyed in areas that might seem impossible to make improvements.

IF and Positive Effects on Periods, Fertility, and Metabolism

Below are a few specific concerns that all women have in regards to attempting new diet plans. How will it affect some of the basic functions of the woman's body and will it be positive? Knowing this information will help you make the decision to start IF sooner than later.

Positive Impacts on Periods

The delicate balance of the hormones in women makes it essential to plan and carry out the IF routine in a gradual increasing way. Throwing yourself into it with reckless abandonment can result in tipping the scales of balance on your hormones. You will experience normal period activity unless you add too much stress from battling carb overload or insulin stimulation.

Reducing stress on the cells of your body is a way of reducing stress on the organs. You'll find your period coming and going on a normal schedule, with less complication and anxiety. You might find that any pre-menstrual symptoms completely disappear

IF and Fertility Improvements

IF can improve fertility naturally by the steady drop in weight that makes you feel better about yourself. You will feel more attractive for your mate, which can lead to increased bedroom activity, resulting in pregnancy.

Fasting is also shown to lessen the presence of cortisol, which can reduce your chances of successful and timely ovulation. Your ovulation schedule will normalize into a recognizable pattern that can be better predicted. When both partners enter fasting windows, the increased fertility grows exponentially.

Picking Up Your Metabolism

Your rate of metabolism determines how fast your body burns fuel for energy to operate the organs, muscles, and use the brain. Ultimately, it determines how fast you can experience permanent weight loss. Dropping weight too fast is a sure sign that you are losing a ton of water out of your system. You can pay for this by ending up suffering dehydration.

IF boosts your metabolic rate in two ways. One is to trigger higher amounts of self-eating or autophagy. The second is to switch your body to burning fat, rather than sugars and carbs in the body. You will see huge weight loss numbers pretty fast. Begin by trying the uncomplicated 12-hour eating window and 12-hour fast and see how you feel.

Being in a state of constant stress can leave you feeling miserable and at risk of illness and disease. It impacts your sleep and ability to get things done. Not reducing stress can lead to anxiety problems, weight gain, or depression. IF can bring you the beneficial changes that help reduce stress.

Defeating Stress and a Feeling of Well-Being

The better you feel on a daily basis, the calmer your day will seem. You can easily maintain an upbeat attitude and fewer things overwhelm you. Maintaining IF and keeping your body free of toxins is an easy way to improve how you feel. Toxins cause illness and a sluggish feel to movements, thoughts, and reactions.

The use of autophagy to clean up the cellular "trash" in your system and improve cell performance will also make you feel better each day. As you deepen the autophagy over extended periods, you will literally begin to turn back time with your cells in some respects. Don't be surprised if you begin to feel some of the energy of your younger years returning. It can slow the aging process without using pills, surgery, lotions, or creams. Natural anti-aging is something money can't buy and brings lasting joy.

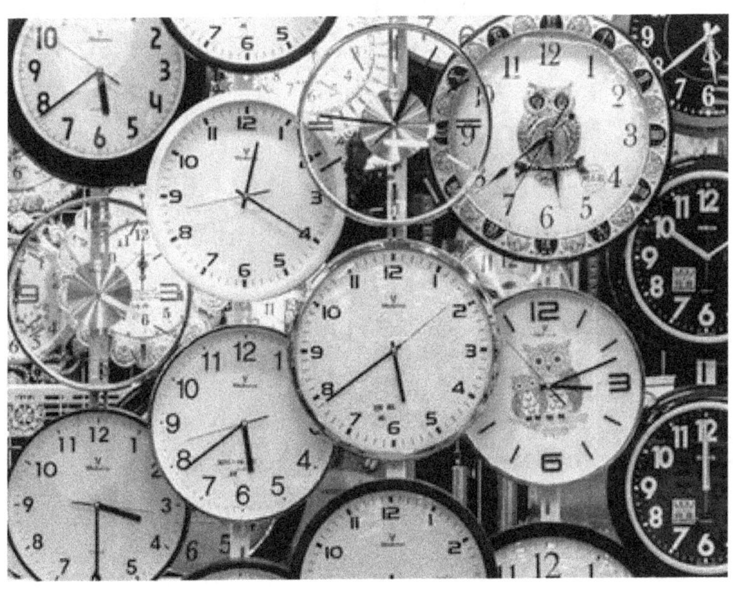

Simplifying Your Schedule

Imagine easing up an already hectic schedule by reducing down to one eating window each day? Fasting for 24 hours every other day can also simplify your schedule. Less meals to fix and worry over gives you extra time to take care of other things. You can begin to lose weight without stressing and worrying about the process. It's a simpler way to take care of your body and enjoy all the benefits IF offers.

Stress and the Brain

Oxidation stressors and a lack of neuroplasticity in the brain that lacks adequate nutrition and is filled with toxins can affect how well you think, function, learn, and behave. The fasting involved in IF gives you a chance to rid the brain of the bad stuff and reduces your chance of early onset of diseases that affect memory, balance, and physical performance. It can melt a ton of stress off your life.

Choose Easy IF Routines When Under Stress

Pick an easier, less complicated IF routine if you are in a period of high-stress. The 12-hour fast and 12-hour eating window is straightforward and easy to keep track of. The Warrior Diet is another IF plan that is simplified and effective. You will begin to notice over time that stress affects you less and less when it comes to handling your IF goals.

Don't feel bad if you feel the need to exit a fast if the stress of daily life has made it too uncomfortable to continue or you begin feeling health problems from the stress of everything. IF is not intended to make life more complicated. Wait until things get sorted out and give it another try.

IF for the Muscle-Building Queen

When your goal is to lean out, cut fat, and increase your muscle mass, careful planning of your IF schedule and workouts must be made and observed. It can be done, but doing it wrong can cost you muscle.

Cutting Calories and Working Out

Planning to build muscle is not easy when using IF, but there is a way to do it safely and comfortably. You can completely balance the food you need and the reduced calories it takes to create leaner, stronger muscles. Lighter calorie days need to incorporate your lighter, toning exercise routines. Exercising on your fast days should be reserved for those that can physically handle it and have a doctor's okay.

Provide What Your Body Needs to Repair and Build Muscle

The preparation for muscle building while on IF has an equal amount to do with intake of the right nutrients and providing the exercise opportunities to break down muscle for repair and building. In other words, you need to eat the foods your body needs to have the energy to work out and you need to do the exercise that's required to provide muscle building.

You'll have to adjust both to accommodate whichever IF plan you choose to begin. Doing too much exercise on your fast days can be detrimental. Not eating enough nutritious food you need can also work against your efforts. Finding a balance that works is essential. The best IF plans to use are the alternating Fast and eat days. You can also try the 12:12 or 16:8, as long as you make sure to increase carbs on the meal right before your work out. Plan your workouts to be between 2 and 3 hours after your meal.

Once your system is used to the 16:8, you can switch to the lean-gains method of restricting calories to what you need to promote new muscle growth. The following chapter gives a better description as to how you go about doing the lean-gains method.

Workouts Before, During, and After the Fast

The designated eating window days should be used for just that — eating. Eat the right mix of foods you need to ensure you are maintaining ketosis, but add the necessary carbs and protein your body needs to repair and build new muscle tissue. Plan your toughest workouts on your eating days. You'll have the access to calories needed to safely perform without feeling weak, dizzy, or a lack of motivation.

Fast days should be spent doing a low activity to avoid burning up valuable muscle tissue. The body will burn anything readily available if you place too many demands for fuel in a fasting state. The eating window following your fasting period allows you to resume your intense work out after putting the nutrition in your system you'll need. Carefully monitoring your diet and activity levels will allow you to lean the muscles you have and build new tissue, as well as drop unneeded pounds of fat.

IF When Breastfeeding

The divide in the opinion of breastfeeding moms doing fasts is loaded with strong opinions on both sides. Many moms experience great results when using IF during breastfeeding. Breast milk has been tested to show higher amounts of fat, which can make the baby feel fuller, longer. It depends on the fasting plan you go with and make sure you follow the best nutritional uptake during the eating window.

As with any dieting plan, discuss IF and the plan you want to use with your doctor and pediatrician. This book is not designed to replace the advice of a qualified physician that understands your particular health needs and that of your baby.

Plan for the Eating Window to Go by the Wayside

It might seem counterintuitive to fast when you are eating to supply two people with fuel and vitamins. In actuality, the body of the woman is designed to store up vitamin, minerals, and fat reserves to sustain life for periods of lack or famine. You need to make the fast periods shorter in duration. Full 24-hour fasting days are too taxing. You won't have enough energy to care for the baby. A 12-

hour fast and 12-hour feast is a simple one that seems to agree with most new moms.

It's never been more important to listen to the cues your body is giving than during your fasting period. If you are feeding the baby heavily and suddenly feel starved, break the fast and eat. If you wake up feeling starved in the morning on your fasting day, eat. Your body is telling you it needs nutrients and you should always listen.

Increase Your Carbs in the First Months

The most demands for nutrients when breastfeeding will be in the first few months. Add at least 100 extra grams of carbs to your diet during each eating window to ensure you have the fuel your body needs for energy. Taking care of a young baby will prove taxing at times and you'll appreciate having the extra source of fuel.

You'll need to add even more carbs as you progress over the months and decide to add any exercise routines to your eating window days. Keep in mind how many avenues you have nutrition being used and drained. Re-adjust as needed based on how you're feeling. Discontinue a fast anytime you aren't feeling healthy and comfortable.

Drink Plenty of Fluids and Get Plenty of Vitamins/Minerals

Drinking fluids and staying hydrated are critical to the health of you and your baby when breastfeeding. Drink if you feel thirsty. Hydration is needed to burn the fuel in your body and to create breast milk. Increase your water intake if your milk level production begins to drop. Add a great multi-vitamin that is safe to ingest when breastfeeding. Check in periodically with your doctor and the pediatrician during your IF progress. Don't shoot for more intensive fasting when breastfeeding. Find a comfortable schedule and wait to get on tougher plans when you're done breastfeeding.

Polycystic Ovary Syndrome is a condition that causes the development of cysts on the ovaries, swelling, hormonal imbalance, and insulin resistance. It's extremely hard for women with PCOS to lose weight. Many are turning to IF and are finding relief and real results. Unfortunately, there are no long-term studies on the benefits of IF and PCOS relief, but most report noticeable results in lessening symptoms and reduced overall stress by following the IF plan faithfully.

PCOS and Hormonal Imbalance

Whatever IF plan you chose should be started gently to avoid even further hormonal imbalance. The 12:12 and 16:8 are great to start with and experiment with to see how your body responds. Most of your fasting time can be as you sleep, which you would normally do.

PCOS causes fertility problems, which is another reason to be mindful of the balance in hormones. Pull back from fasting if you begin to suffer unexpected mood swings or constantly changing internal temperatures. It signals a major fluctuation in hormones. The slower you start, the less noticeable it will be.

PCOS and Insulin Resistance

Insulin resistance is a condition in which the cells are unable to utilize the hormone insulin, produced by the pancreas, effectively to burn glucose for fuel. The glucose stays in the bloodstream at high levels, indicating a prediabetes condition. PCOS sufferers are more likely to deal with insulin resistance on a consistent basis.

IF is shown to reduce insulin resistance when coupled with a ketogenic diet. The cell repair and healing of autophagy has everything to do with getting many cases of insulin resistance under control. It can back you down off the ledge of diabetes.

Lose Weight and Reduce Stress with IF

Two of the biggest struggles for those with PCOS are the inability to lose stubborn fat and the high levels of stress in not knowing when to expect the next round of health problems. It seems as if life is lived from one doctor visit to the next. You can break free of this by putting yourself on an IF plan that's easy and gives you real results.

Weight loss will benefit you be reducing all of the symptoms associated with PCOS and you'll feel better. As symptoms subside, the stress will begin to melt away. Life will begin to reach a semblance of normal. You will find that doctor visits get fewer and farther between.

IF for Mature or Menopausal Women

The menopausal and post-menopausal woman is sensitive to the slightest changes in hormone levels and can undergo severe symptoms if everything gets out of balance. You must introduce IF gradually and slowly expand your fasting window, but never exceed 16 hours total fasting at one time. You can begin with the 12:12 and gradually expand to 16:8 as your body and symptoms allow.

Hot Flashes and Night Sweats

The expected fluctuations in hormones can make it difficult to sleep with hot flashes and night sweats. As your body gets used to the fasting periods and the hormones begin to get more balanced, the symptoms will lessen. You can also try drinking water only in the evening. It helps to keep these types of symptoms at bay.

If you feel that the hormone raging has worsened, back off on the plan or end the fast. Revisit your diet intake during the eating windows. Make sure you are taking in enough nutrition and are not packing it with sugars or carbs.

Post-Menopausal Weight Gains

Weight gain is one of the top complaints of post-menopausal women. It seems to gather up in the mid-section and not want to leave, no matter how much you exercise. IF shines in being able to get rid of post-menopausal weight in a permanent way. You'll want to make it a way of life. Increasing the ability of your slowing metabolism to burn fat instead of carbs is a sensible way to break the trend of steadily increasing body weight. Once you are set at the 16-hour fasting state and 8-hour eating window, you can begin trying to incorporate the 5:2 plan that has you eating 500 calories or less during your eating window.

Remove Nighttime Sugars, Caffeine, and Alcohol

The battle for sleep and fluctuating anxiety levels can last for years when going through and leaving the menopausal time period. The best thing you can do as you use the IF pan is to eliminate the use of sugars, caffeine, and alcohol past 6 pm during your eating windows. You will have less sustained insulin activity and the caffeine will not interfere with your sleep or cause nervousness and fidgeting. You'll end the tossing and turning that accompanies the inability to sleep.

Ghrelin and Leptin

One thing that works against diet success for mature and menopausal women is the sudden surge in the hormones, ghrelin and leptin. These two are responsible for those intense hunger pangs you feel that make your stomach rumble so bad it can seemingly be picked up by seismograph machines. The imbalance of hormones means your system will be releasing more of these particular hormones. You will feel hungry all the time and it's hard to break the mental connect. It's one reason why you need to start slow and work up gradually with an IF plan. Break the fast and eat low-calorie if you must.

Chapter 4: Types of IF Diets

The type of IF diet you choose will help determine how successful your first try is and whether you want to continue. It's always best to start light and increase as your mind and body gets used to what fasting is all about. This chapter will give you all the details you need on what each type consists of and how it can work with your work and personal schedule, the benefits, and what problems might arise. You can make a more informed choice on which is best to start.

Crescendo Method

The crescendo method of fasting is blending two or three days of 12 to 16-hour fasts on different days of the week. Keep at least one regular diet day between each day of fasting. It is not as regimented as some IF plans and can give you great results without a ton of effort. You must be careful in how you plan the diet around work and home life.

Benefits of the Crescendo Method

- Gain increasing experience at fasting for longer and longer periods of time.
- Less mental and physical stress with days of a normal diet in between fasts.
- Increased autophagy and body toxin cleansing.
- Increased fat burning when done routinely.
- Less chance of hormone imbalance due to short duration and regular meal days between.
- You can stick with this plan for weeks as you gradually increase your fasting times.

How to do the Crescendo Method

You need to first decide if you are going to attempt a clean fast or you will allow yourself extremely low-calorie beverages during the fast state. Eat well the day before your fast and begin counting time from your last meal of the night before. Do not eat anything else until your designated time period has elapsed. You can then eat normally for your eating window.

What it Looks Like

Here is a sample of what the crescendo method schedule would look like if you chose to fast 3 days for 12 hours per fast state. We'll choose Monday, Wednesday, and Friday as the fast days for this example:

Sunday: Begin counting your fast time for the Monday start at the end of your last meal on Sunday. Make sure you do not take in any other calories. Let's place your evening meals at 6 pm for easy calculating.

Monday: Actual fast lasts from 7 pm Sunday (allowing for one hour to eat the meal) and you will not eat again until 7 am. 14-hour fasting paces the eating window starting at 9 am. The 16-hour fast places the window at 11 am.

Tuesday: Normal meals with the final meal finished by 5 pm.

Wednesday: If you have to get up and ready for work earlier than 7 am, you can adjust your last mealtime for the evening before. Moving it back to 5 pm places the start of your eating window at 5 am for the 12-hour fast, 7 am for the 14-hour fast, and 9 am for the 16-hour fast.

Thursday: Normal meals with the final meal of the day finished by 3 pm.

Friday: If you have to get up even earlier and want to eat a hearty breakfast, back the finish of your last meal the night before by the appropriate number of hours. A finish time of 3 pm the night before places the eating window start at 3 am for the 12-hour fast, 5 am for the 14-hour fast, and 7 am for the 16-hour fast.

Saturday: Normal meals.

Potential Problems

The only potential problems with this fasting method are that it can interfere with evening events like business dinners, anniversary celebrations, or family gatherings involving food. You can always switch up the days of the week as long as you make sure to place one regular meal day between the fasting days.

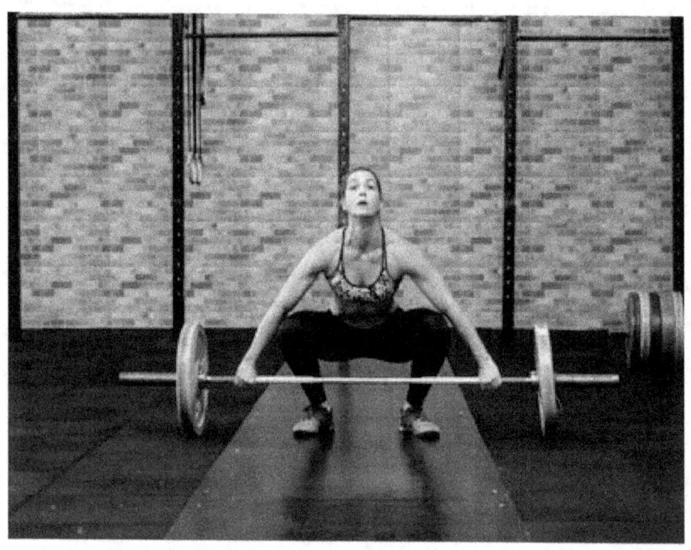

Lean-Gains Method

The lean-gains IF method is one that combines strict fasting and controlled calorie intake to combine the best in leaning out your existing muscle and building more. You will alternate from the largest meal after the fast being the last on workout days and first on resting days. Your total calorie intake should be 20 calories for every pound of weight. For a 130-pound woman, the daily calorie intake should be 130 X 20 calories = 2600 calories. Work out days needs to have more than the 5 percent carbs recommended. Protein should always rest at about 30 percent and the remainder as healthy fat. Incorporate at least three doses of BCAA amino acid mixture per day.

Benefits of Lean-Gains

- Greater control over calories in your diet.
- The ultimate way to lean your muscle and expand muscle tissue.
- Easy to fast during the way to fast through partial working hours and hit the gym after work.
- Extreme increase in metabolic rate and fat burning.
- Extending fast into morning makes it more social-friendly for evening planning.

How to do Lean Gains

You begin lean-gains by starting a standard 16:8 IF plan. Choose how many days per week you want to fast and work out. The remainder will be normal, resting days. Calculate your suggested calorie intake using the formula above. Divide your smallest meals into 25 percent of your daily calories each. A 10 to 15 percent calorie intake snack and the remainder for the large meal of the day. The large meal is first on resting days and lasts on work out days.

What it Looks Like

Sunday: Large meal first, Small meal, snack, small meal finished by 7 pm. Start fasting.

Monday: Eating window starts at 3 pm. Small meal first, snack, small meal, work out, large meal.

Tuesday: Large meal, small meal, snack, small meal, finish and start fast at 7 pm.

Wednesday: Start eating window at 3 pm. Small meal, snack, small meal, workout, large meal.

Thursday: Large meal, small meal, snack, small meal, finish last meal by 7 pm and start fasting.

Friday: Eating window start at 7 am. Small meal, small meal, snack, work out, large meal.

Saturday: Large meal, small meal, snack, small meal, and remain off fast until Sunday.

Potential Problems

You may find that you are taking in the wrong mix of foods or too many calories, resulting in increased fat storage. It's expensive and difficult to stay on such a highly-restrictive diet. Cheating on the fast is a possibility.

16:8 Fasting

16:8 fasting is a versatile method that can be used to go an intense 16 hours or back off and stick with a medium level of 12 to 14 hours of fasting. The majority of the fast can be done as you sleep. You can finish the fast during the morning hours and simply skip breakfast on your way to work.

Benefits of 16:8 Fasting

- Natural way to fast that uses the innate tendency to skip breakfast in the mornings.
- Easily adjusts to make it more intense.
- Can use in conjunction with other fasting like 5:2 and lean-gains.
- Good, solid fast that produces positive fat burning results fast.
- Easy to fit with your work or play schedule by changing days or adjusting start times for fasting.

How to do 16:8 Fasting

Start out by doing 12:12 or 14:10 before moving on the 16:8. 16 hours of fasting can seem like a long time if you are not familiar with how it can make you feel. You can ease the impact to your system by gradually stepping up your fasting hours, rather than plunging headlong into 16 hours. The fast is followed by an 8-hour window of eating. You can fit two medium size meals or three small ones easily into an 8-hour period.

What it Looks Like

Once again, we'll pretend that someone is fasting Monday, Wednesday, and Friday. The schedule will look like this:

Sunday: Normal meals with the last one at ending at 7 pm. Start fasting.

Monday: End fast at 7 am with an eating window of 12 hours or 7 pm. The eating window is until 9 pm for 14-hour fasting and 11 pm for 16-hour fasting.

Tuesday: Normal meals and end at eating at 5 pm if you want an earlier eating window to fit with work or outside activities.

Wednesday: Eating window starts at 5 am for 12-hour fasting, 7 am for 14-hour, and 9 am for 16-hour fast.

Thursday: Normal meals and we will back up the last meal to end at 3 pm if you need an even earlier start to your eating window.

Friday: Eating window starts at 3 am for 12-hour fasting, 5 am for 14-hour fasting, and 7 am for the full 16-hour fast.

Saturday: Normal meals and no fasting.

Possible Problems

16 hours is a long time to go without food and if you don't properly hydrate and take in nourishment during your eating window, your blood sugar level can drop. It can drop quickly if you are eating too many carbs during your fed state. Exit the fast and try again on your next fast date after fixing the diet. Take your time and work up to the 16 hours over time. It may not be an appropriate method for those already experiencing extreme hormonal fluctuations.

The 20:4 method or Warrior Diet is one that's perfectly designed for the high-energy, once a day eater. You won't even realize you're on a fasting regimen other than blocking out snacks and calorie-filled drinks as you fast. It's about as intense as it gets for a daily fast, but you also have a window of opportunity for food every day.

Benefits of the Warrior Diet

- Fairly no-maintenance fasting routine almost anyone can do.
- Similar to days when you're too busy to eat until you get home from work.
- Perfect for people that like to go out to eat in the evening.
- Easily adjust start and stop times to fit your work and off-time schedule.

How to do the Warrior Diet

The Warrior Diet isn't hard to master. You drink water and non-calorie drinks for your full 20-hour fasting period and squeeze your nutritional needs into a four-hour window at the end of your day. You can typically fit in a decent meal and a snack. It's the preferred method of eating for many busy people. The changes you make to carb intake will make a huge difference in your fat burning

What it Looks Like

We use the Mon, Tues, Wed, Thurs, and Fri routine for this fasting method. You need to think ahead as to the time you would prefer the eating window to begin. It can be based on an upcoming event with food or the time it takes to get home from work.

Sunday: Normal meals to start. The last meal should end at 7 pm if you want your eating window to start earlier.

Monday: Fast all day until 3 pm when the eating window opens. End eating by 7 pm. Start fasting again.

Tuesday: Fast until 3 pm and eat until 7 pm. Start fast again.

Wednesday: Fast until 3 pm and eat until 7 pm. Start fast again.

Thursday: Fast until 3 pm and eat until 7 pm. Start fast again.

Friday: Fast until 3 pm and eat as normal.

Saturday: Normal meals.

Possible Problems

Most people don't realize what their overall calorie intake is every day. You are often eating without being aware of it. Grabbing a cookie in the office, a snack out of the vending machine, or hot dog off the vending cart can all go unnoticed when you're fasting. You might even grab a fruit juice if you begin to feel your energy sapped. None of that can happen during your fast. You do risk falling off the fasting wagon during the day.

12:12 fasting is one of the simplest IF plans there is to follow. You split your day in half. One part is complete fast and the other is your eating window. It's a fast you can easily do every day and make it a dietary lifestyle change. The calories you will remove from your diet and increased metabolism will help you stay at a healthy weight.

Benefits of 12:12 Fasting

- The eating window is as long as the fasting window.
- Comfortable eating window that allows for full meals.
- Most of the fasting is done at night, which limits uncomfortable feelings of hunger.
- Adjustable to fit a working schedule or busy evening social life.
- Lessens feelings of food deprivation.

How to do 12:12 Fasting

You begin your fast the night before. Set it at a time that is comfortable for ending the eating window the next day. If you enjoy a snack in the evening, wait until around 7 pm to start the fast. You will then have from 7 am to 7 pm the next day to eat.

What it Looks Like

We will use every day on this list to carry out the 12:12 diet, as many people prefer to do this one daily.

Sunday: Eat normal meals but begin fast at 7 pm.

Monday: End fast at 7 am. Eat a hearty breakfast before work. Finish eating for the day by 7 pm. Begin fasting.

Tuesday: End fast at 7 am with a good breakfast. End eating for the day at 7 pm. Begin fasting again.

Wednesday: End fast at 7 am. Eat normal meals but begin fast again at 7 pm.

Thursday: End fast and begin eating window at 7 am. Eat normal meals and resume fasting at 7 pm.

Friday: Begin eating window at 7 am. Eat normally throughout the day and resume fast at 7 pm.

Saturday: End fasting at 7 am and eat normally through the day. Either begin fasting again at 7 pm or exit IF plan.

Possible Problems

The 12:12 plan can be hard for someone that prefers to eat snacks at night. You have to fit your eating during the day primarily, which can be difficult if you work long hours. You might have to adjust the start times to better fit your work hours and availability to get the nutrition you need to stay healthy and satisfied. You might have trouble with hunger pangs at night. If so, drink a cup of clear broth to get you through until morning. Avoid midnight snacking at all costs.

The randomness of spontaneous skipping might be a fun way for you to begin venturing into the world of IF plans and methods. Most people using the spontaneous skipping method pick random meals to skip 3 or 4 days each week. It's the perfect way to test the waters and get the feel for how your body reacts to fasting. It's the easiest IF method to use at work and at home.

Benefits of Spontaneous Skipping

- You are in control of when to eat and when to skip a meal.
- No long fast for a more comfortable experience.

- Excellent starter method for IF.
- Great way to reduce calories without officially "dieting."
- Begin a steady detox and cleansing of your body.

How to do Spontaneous Skipping

All that's involved with spontaneous skipping is to decide which days you want to concentrate on and then choose which meal to skip. You have complete flexibility, which makes it easier for those moments you are spontaneously asked out to lunch or dinner. You can skip the next meal instead.

What it Looks Like

We'll pretend that the individual is skipping one meal on Mon, Wed, and Fri. The schedule will look similar to this, although any meal on those days can be skipped.

Sunday: Normal meals.

Monday: Skip breakfast, water, and unsweetened, non-calorie drinks until lunch. Normal meals for the rest of the day.

Tuesday: Normal Meals.

Wednesday: Normal breakfast, Normal lunch, no food after lunch and skip dinner. Fast until next morning.

Thursday: Normal meals.

Friday: Normal breakfast, no snacking after breakfast, and skip lunch. Normal dinner.

Saturday: Normal meals.

Possible Problems

It's tempting to move a meal up sooner if you begin having hunger pangs. Avoid this and zero snacking when skipping a meal.

The eat-skip-eat method is one that alternates full meal days of normal eating with a 24-hour fast in between. It is generally done once or twice a week. It's another simpler form of IF that is easier to put into a busy schedule without much planning or thought. You will want to try a few of the skip meal days first to get the feel for what you might be getting into.

Benefits of Skip-Eat-Skip Method

- Great for busy days and ones that are stay-at-home lazy days. You will either be too busy to notice or can sleep your way through the worst of the fasting period.
- You get the full benefit of 24-hours of toxin cleansing and metabolism boosting.
- You can exit the fast if there is a problem and try again without a long wait.

How to do Skip-Eat-Skip Method

You need to start your fast the evening before. Count the time from the last meal forward. You will enter your eating window exactly 24 hours from the time you start. In 24 more hours, you restart the fast. 24 hours after this, you can eat normally.

What it Looks Like

We will show what a schedule looks like for someone choosing to eat-skip-eat on Sunday through Tuesday and again on Wednesday through Friday of the same week. The schedule will look similar to this:

Sunday: Normal meals until Sunday evening. Begin the fast at 6 pm (or at the end of your last meal.)

Monday: Continue fast until 24 hours after you began the fast. At 6 pm, you can begin enjoying normal meals.

Tuesday: Normal meals.

Wednesday: Normal meals until 6 pm. Begin 24 hour fast.

Thursday: Continue fast until 6 pm. Enjoy normal meals again.
Friday: Normal meals.

Saturday: Normal meals.

Possible Problems

A 24-hour long fast is a long time to go without a snack or calorie-filled drink. You can get used to it, but it's best to start gradually. Your biggest problems could range from feeling fatigue from lack of quick energy carbs or hunger pangs from missing meals you are used to eating. It's hard to avoid the temptation to snack so be prepared to tell yourself not to take the plunge.

5:2 Fasting

The 5:2 fasting method is a flexible way to cut down on calories a couple of days a week without doing a complete fast. It's considered a modified fasting method that works to increase your metabolism and make you less insulin resistant. It's the perfect IF plan for anyone that cannot do the complete fasting due to irregular hormone outputs or medication issues.

Benefits of 5:2 Fasting

- Flexible choice on days of the week to do modified fasting.
- Easy to fast with limited calories when you need to take prescribed medications with food.
- Less hunger pangs.
- Appreciable toxin cleansing and metabolism boost.

How to do 5:2 Fasting

Choose two non-consecutive days to do your modified fasting. Pick the foods and drinks you want for that day that amount to 500 to 800 total calories. Plan the best times to take in these calories. Try a light snack for midday and a light dinner for the best results in fighting back hunger. The fast for your chosen day will begin after the last meal on the day before. It will end exactly 24 hours later. You get maximum fasting benefits by starting the process later in the evening.

What it Looks Like

We will choose Monday and Friday as the modified fasting days. The schedule will look similar to this:

Sunday: Normal meals but begin fast at 9 pm.

Monday: Skip breakfast and eat a low-calorie brunch. Eat a small, low-calorie dinner. Stop at your desired calorie limit and no more food after 9 pm. Technically the fast is over but going to bed without eating anything more that day will help boost the effectiveness.

Tuesday: Normal meals.

Wednesday: Normal meals.

Thursday: Normal meals but start fasting at 9 pm.

Friday: Light breakfast or brunch. Small, low-calorie dinner that is finished by 9 pm. Go to bed without eating anything further that day.

Saturday: Normal meals.

Possible Problems

You can adjust your calories to meet your nutritional needs but try to avoid binge eating. You might do fine until evening and have a hard time limiting calories further. Add a cup of warm broth if you still feel hungry. This is a plan that should work well with almost any job schedule.

Alternate Day Fasting

Alternating your fasting and eating days is another way to get maximum health benefits and weight loss without feeling totally deprived of the foods you love. You can do this 2 or 3 days each week and enjoy terrific benefits. It's the perfect type of fasting for those that want to get serious about weight loss, metabolism boosting, complete cleansing, and safely do strenuous exercises for the fed state days.

Benefits of Alternate Day Fasting

- You get a complete rest from fasting every 24 hours.
- You can restart the fasting the next day if you goof up and break the fast.
- Perfect for those maintaining rigorous workout routines.
- Less chance of hormonal imbalances with limited fasting.

How to do Alternate Day Fasting

Choose your days for complete 24-hour fasts. Maintain one day between each fasting day as one with normal meals. Begin your fast on the evening of the day before, right after your last meal.

What it Looks Like

Let's pretend that someone is starting an alternating day fast and has chosen Monday, Wednesday, and Friday as the complete fasting days. The schedule will look similar to this:

Sunday: Normal meals but begin fasting at 7 pm.

Monday: Complete fast until 7 pm. You can eat a small meal at this point but try not to overeat.

Tuesday: Normal meals until 7 pm when you restart the fasting.

Wednesday: Continue fast until 7 pm. Eat small calories.

Thursday: Normal meals until fasting restarts at 7 pm.

Friday: Continue fasting until 7 pm. Eat a small dinner or snack and call it a day.

Saturday: Normal meals.

Possible Problems

The biggest problems you are likely to encounter with this IF plan is the urge to binge-eat at the end of your fast. It can prove a taxing method if you do strenuous activities at work. You may have to drop down to a modified, low-calorie version. Try and keep your weekends free where you can catch up on healthy, nutritious eating.

You can modify these various IF methods and plans to fit your needs and increase in the intensity of fasting as you move through and get used to the fasting experience. Keep in tune with how you are feeling and your body responds. Make any adjustments that are needed. Exit the fast any time you feel uncomfortable or something doesn't feel quite right. Make your first meal soft foods or broth if you have been fasting close to 24 hours to avoid stomach upset.

Chapter 5: The 14-Day Pyramid-Fasting Process to a Slimmer You

Now it's time to take all of the information you've learned about IF and create a perfect, customized plan you can start right away. This chapter will explain how to choose the right plan and adjust it to fit your exact needs and get the results you want. All you need is the right plan and the right preparation to begin losing weight and feeling better for the rest of your life!

Customizing the Process to Your Needs

All of the concentrated thinking you did in Chapter 2 about what motivated you to try intermittent fasting applies at this point. Gather up any notes you took and keep them handy as you go through the process of choosing an IF plan that meets your motivational and physical needs.

What are some of the plans that you found interesting or easy enough to try? Each one will require some level of customization to fit your exact lifestyle and level of available time. It's best to pick one starting program with an eye on the second one to level up to after a two-week period. Always staying in forward motion will propel you towards success.

Focus on Your Motivation

What is it that is motivating you to try IF? Are you looking to drop weight? Are you worried about your blood sugar levels? Are you wanting to jumpstart your battle against cellular aging? Have you entered menopause and notice that metabolism is slowing down? IF plans are available that can answer nearly any health and wellness concern.

Making the best choice takes looking at the mechanics of what you want to accomplish. Developing leaner muscles will require a more rigorous fasting routine that allows for periods of eating to pack in the healthy nutrients that are essential for muscular growth and leaning. Boosting metabolism can be done at every level of IF. Even the less stringent fasting routines allow for reduced insulin resistance and faster metabolism.

Stop what you are doing right now and write down at least two IF plans that sound easy enough to start with and add a secondary one that's a little tougher to switch to after your first two-week

Adapting an IF Plan

The IF plan you choose to start with can be fully customized and modified to fit your life and your goals. Not everyone works on the same days or the same hours. Not everyone does the same activities after work or enjoys the same time off. You can address all of the specifics and work out the details to fit your schedule to an amazing degree.

For the rest of this chapter, we will pretend that you have chosen the 12:12 plan with the eventual stepping up to 16:8. The first order of business is to decide what day of the week you want to start your plan in action. Would it be better to start on a day off from work, or have work as the distraction for your first fasting day?

Fasting Start/Stop

The next step in customizing your IF plan is to determine the right time of the day to start your fasting period. It partially is determined by the outcome you want in resulting eating window, but you might have that last comfort snack of the evening in mind that you aren't prepared to give up. Starting at 7 pm at night will give you an ending time of 7 am for the 12-hour fast and graduate out to 11 am for the full 16-hour fast you intend to expand towards.

What is the normal time you have your last meal or snack in the evening? Can you modify this to adjust to a two or three day fast during the week? Read the next section before setting a time in stone. Both must be equally considered to devise the right plan for you.

Eating Window Start/Stop

If you decide to fast on your day off, the start of the eating window might not matter. If you begin on a workday, are you in need of being able to eat breakfast before heading out the door? The ending time of the fast will become an important thing to keep in mind if you have to leave your house before the eating window begins. You can adjust the start time back to accommodate or pack a breakfast to take with you and eat when you are entering the eating window.

Low or No-Calorie Fasting

Make the decision before you start as to whether your fasting periods will be clean or completely zero calories. You can modify the fast to include low-calorie things like broth, coffee creamer (almond mild or similar low-calorie product), and a twist of lemon or lime to your water. You may not need this at a 12-hour fasting rate but it might be good to keep in mind as you expand it to 16-hours.

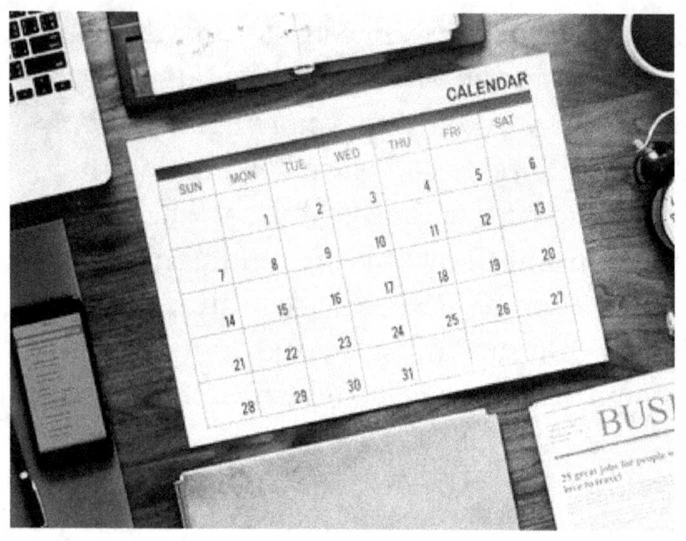

Shifting with Work Schedules

The 12:12 and 16:8 fasting methods can be moved and shifted to accommodate any changes to your work schedule. It's important if you work in a business that doesn't maintain the same schedule all the time. Take a look at the upcoming schedule and move the fast to meet your new days off or the days of your choice. Make sure you don't place the fasting days back-to-back. You can expand to doing more fast days as you get used to fasting, but don't push yourself too hard when starting out.

Shifting with Personal Schedules

You may not have to completely change fasting days if you are looking at starting your fast on an evening that coincides with a business or personal dinner engagement, family holiday, or other evening food-involved event. If eating extends past your normal start time, push it a little later and end the fast the requisite number of hours the next day. It might mean a longer delay in being able to eat the next day, but your fasting will still be on track.

Transitioning to IF

Transitioning to IF can be a complete shock to your body if you are eating an unhealthy diet and in unbalanced proportions. Focus on ways to clean up your act before you start your IF plan. All the efforts you make in this area will be beneficial and add to your success. Spend at least two weeks making the switches and changes you need to feel confident and ready to start IF. The first thing you need to do is take a close look at what your current diet is like. You might be surprised at how much needs to change.

Discover Your Basic Eating Habits

Spend one day completely documenting personal eating and drinking habits. It doesn't have to include calorie counts or anything that specific, but include everything down to a piece of gum. Most people are shocked by how much food they freely consume in a 24-hour period. It can point to what some of your weaknesses are, as far as diet and times of day you prefer to snack. Those will be the danger points to avoid when starting your fasting routine.

Documenting one day is all you need to get a baseline, as long as it's a normal day and you don't purposefully avoid things knowing you are documenting the experience. It's nothing that will be shown to others. It's for your own edification. What you are looking for is signatures of unhealthy eating patterns and attractions to unhealthy foods. Those will be your biggest struggles.

Learn to Listen to Your Body

Your body is good at giving clues on how it's handling stress and whether anything is happening health-wise that needs monitoring. It pays to be mindful and recognize the often-subtle signals. The more you are in tune with your body communication, the better you'll be at knowing when and how to adjust your IF plan for comfort, safety, and success.

If your moods begin to become a complete roller coaster experience, back off slightly on the fasting or switch to a low-calorie intake fast for a couple of weeks. It's your body signaling that your hormones are coming out of balance. Learn to recognize physical symptoms like headaches, weakness, extreme hunger pains, and dizziness. You should discontinue your fast if these symptoms are noticeable and lasting.

Everyone's experience with fasting differs and each time can bring a new level of difficulties or successes. Make sure you feel comfortable with the level of fasting you are on before expanding or using a more intense approach.

Develop Healthy Eating Habits

Switching to healthier eating and eating patterns will prove beneficial your entire life. Losing the urge to grab quick microwave foods or fast food is doing your entire body a favor. Looking at the ingredients list and putting things back that are packed with unsavory materials is another way to help your body. If it has ingredients with names longer than the packaging or completely unpronounceable, it's probably a preservative that's harmful to your system. Go with more organic, natural choices. A few things to avoid are:

- Highly processed foods
- High sugar content
- Non-grass-fed meats
- Heavy starch content
- Triglyceride and complex oils

Fix as many simple, organic meals at home as possible. Home cooked food is usually always more nutritious than anything you can eat at even the best restaurants.

Get Bad and Unhealthy Foods Out of Your House

What are the foods you will have a hard time avoiding when fasting or trying to eat healthier? How much of this lurks in your home? Take time to go through your cupboards, freezer, and refrigerator to clear these items out. Replace them with more acceptable and healthy items for eating and snacking.

Invest in some cookbooks that are packed with healthy meal and snack ideas. Always buy fresh ingredients for better nutritional value. Avoid canned vegetables and fruits that are emptied of much of their value.

Getting the Process Started

You are close to being able to start your IF plan. Only a few more details need to be managed before start day. The better and more thoroughly you prepare, the higher the chances are you won't experience anything negative. Check and double check that the IF plan you've chosen is one that's reasonable and you've made the right adjustments to feel comfortable.

Tips if you've Never Fasted

Being new to fasting can make it seem like a huge mountain to climb. Starting with an easier plan is a more sensible way to go when you are new to fasting routines. You have no idea how your body will react, although you shouldn't have time for anything too serious to go wrong with one of the easier fasts. Here are a few tips to help your first fast seem more comfortable:

- Make sure you know how much water you normally drink during the day. Keep plenty on hand but don't fill your stomach to try and ward off hunger pangs.
- Try a few random days of skipping a meal here and there to see how fasting feels from the light end.

- Understand that 12 hours is not enough time to starve to death. You can make it!
- Only exit the fast if you absolutely need to for health reasons or due to excessive hunger pangs. Many times, slight issues can be pushed through as a challenge. You know your body better than anyone. Exercise good judgment.

Getting the Prep Work Done

Prepare everything in your environment to be ready for your IF plan to start. You don't want to start your fasting routine and find out you don't have the things on hand you need. A few things to keep in mind and have on hand are:

- Have cold, filtered drinking water available at home and in your vehicle.
- Have coffee and a selection of unsweetened teas at the ready for drinking.
- Fix any lunch you are taking to work with you the night before, prior to the start of your fast to avoid weakening and cheating.

- Keep a selection of chicken, beef, and vegetable broth available if you struggle with the fast.

Picking Your Start Date

All that's left is to pick your starting date and mark it on the calendar. Plan it far enough in advance you can properly prepare, but not so far that you forget or get cold feet. 2-weeks maximum from being physically ready is your target start date. The rest of your time should be spent getting emotionally and mentally ready.

Avoid listening to horror stories about fasting and reading fear-porn that can shake your confidence. Read uplifting information. Your chances of anything major going wrong are almost non-existent. Your first fast will be light and short. As long as you are in reasonably good health, you should have a successful start. Set your two-week schedule ahead, if possible.

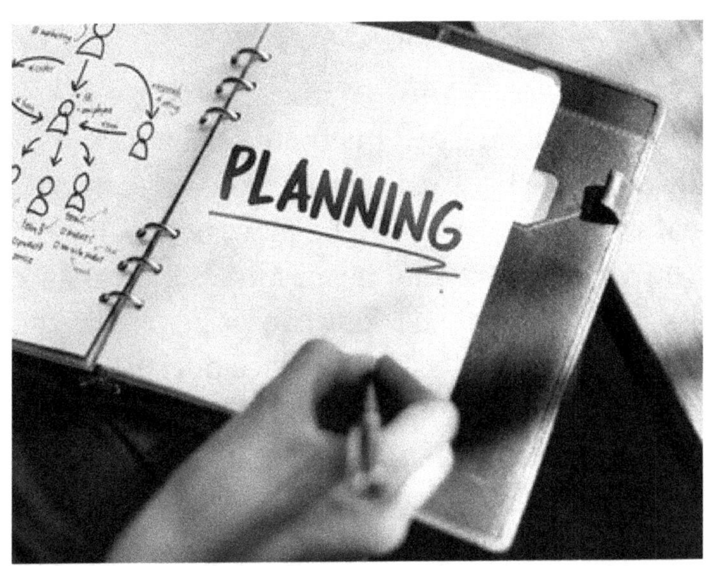

Make Everyone Aware of Your IF Plans

You will have very few problems if you live on your own, but make sure everyone in your household knows of your IF plan before starting. If potato chips are your weakness, prior knowledge can make it easier for those types of foods to not be eaten right in front of you. Not everyone will understand that fasting means staying completely away from calories. Don't make an assumption that you can be strong enough to avoid temptation at the last minute. It could end your fasting quicker than imagined.

The way you feel will fluctuate as you move through the two-week phase of fasting and eating. Your fasting will be more noticeable if you are someone that never misses a meal and likes a late-night snack or two. It helps that the majority of your fast takes place during your sleeping hours. You can still expect a few effects that can change as you move along over the two weeks.

What to Expect Physically

Depending on when you eat dinner in comparison to your fast start time and your bedtime, you might feel rumbles in your tummy as you go to bed. Many people are used to grabbing a snack before bed, especially if dinner ends in the 6 pm range. If you wait to go to bed at 10 pm, you can expect some belly noise the first time or two.

You will feel noticeably famished when you get up the next day and will probably experience the same thing on your second fast day. If you are up at 6 am and have to wait until 7 am to eat, it could be a long hour wait. Once the time passes, you can eat breakfast.

The second week should be a little better. You'll learn to adjust your last meal to include filling items that keep your belly fuller, longer. You might not even realize that the time has gone by in the morning and you can eat. It will get a little more challenging as you spread the fast out later in the day.

What to Expect Mentally

You should feel extremely motivated at the start and finish of your first fast. You'll feel happy at the beginning of the first eating window knowing you were successfully able to avoid cheating. The second fasting day is a little tougher to enter into mentally, especially if you experienced any big level of hunger pangs the first time. It can also be hard to sleep when anticipating the end of the fast.

It becomes more mentally challenging when you expand the fast and you spend more of your awake time struggling with hunger pangs.

At a 14-hour fast, you'll be waiting to eat until 9 am if you start at 7 pm the previous evening. A 16-hour fast will have you skipping breakfast completely and eating at lunchtime. You will begin to find that you're watching the time closely for your first few fasts. The great thing about starting with a 12-hour fast is that you rarely have too many problems in the first two weeks.

Check in with Your Body as You Progress

How are you feeling physically after your first fast? Did you make it through without any jitters or headache? Did you drink enough water to stay hydrated? Try not to drink too much water before bed or you'll be woken unnecessarily to go to the bathroom. You might have a hard time getting back to sleep. Only drink at night if you feel thirsty.

Take note if you experience any problems that are easily resolved by changing your mealtimes, food type, or activity level. Sleep problems are often due to anxiety, too many carbs, or caffeine intake. All of this can be adjusted.

What is Your Energy Level Like?

You should feel plenty of energy the morning after your first fast. You will feel slightly anxious to eat, but the energy levels should be high. The energy level after your first 14-hour fast will be slightly different. You might feel a little jittery on your first morning, but the second should only leave you feeling really hungry.

The first 16-hour fast will be different. You will be used to fasting for 14 hours at a time, but the difference of two hours can be tremendous. Your energy level can drop suddenly at the 9 am timeframe and you'll feel tired until eating at 11 am. This tired feeling tends to go away after two full weeks of 16-hour fasting. Your energy levels return to normal quickly. Reducing carbs on your resting days can sometimes help alleviate this problem.

How to Avoid Cheating

Chapter 7 will contain many ideas to help you avoid cheating and falling off your fasting wagon. If you haven't properly prepared for your fast period, drop back and have a cup of broth and see if that helps you keep going. If that doesn't seem to help, drop back and try a fast with restricted calories until you get used to fasting. Stay away from foods and beverages you have a weakness or predisposition to ingest.

The Value of Journaling

Keep a journal during your fasting experience. It's essential to log everything from how you feel, your energy levels, motivations, and if you are experiencing any problems. Be specific in your descriptions. Also, log moments that you feel great and describe those in detail. Is your thinking clearer? Do you feel more energetic? Is your appetite improved? Are you less focused on food?

Revisit all of your notes each week and see if there is anything you can do to improve your fasting experience. Continue with this process for every week you use an IF plan.

Making Necessary Adjustments

Make sure you are set to go with the next week and that no adjustments need to be made in timing, meal times, length of fast, or any other detail. Try and maintain a healthy diet on the resting days between the fast. Falling back into old, bad eating habits will make the fasting harder. It can set you up for experiencing unpleasant symptoms of fluctuating blood sugar and more.

Climbing Up the Steps

Congratulations for making it through your first two-week IF fasting plan! As with any pyramid, it's time to start climbing to the top. This is one part of the book you may have to revisit each time you decide you want to climb a little higher. It's critical to make sure you are comfortable with the level you are at currently and aren't experiencing any difficulties with the plan. If the answer is positive, proceed to picking your next plan.

Choosing Your Next IF Level Plan

In this chapter, the beginning plan was the 12:12. Doing this for two weeks should be a breeze for nearly anyone. You may want to peruse the choices in plans before making the final decision, but for the purposes of this chapter, let's go with the 16:8 plan. Pull out all of your notes for the last plan and read through them thoroughly. Make sure that any problems are addressed and that you can safely move forward with a slightly more intensive plan.

Transitioning to Your New Plan

In this case, the 16:8 plan is not much different than the 12:12. Had you switched to an alternating day fast, the scheduling and planning would be more extensive. You will have to consider whether any scheduling changes need made for the new 16:8 plan. Is a 7 pm start time going to work? If you favor having a bite to eat before going to work, you might have to back the starting plan up the day before. Finishing your eating by 3 pm might not be possible if you work that day past the time allotted.

The full 16-hour fast typically means that you'll have to give up breakfast. It's easier to stick with a 7 or 8 pm fast starting time and waiting to start your eating window for lunch the next day. It's where the mental difficulties can begin and you start to feel deprived at times. Your mind might remain focused on food for the first week and you are tempted by every fast food driveway you pass. Keep going and head on to work without falling off the fasting wagon. The urges will pass.

The 16:8 plan is not that difficult for someone that is used to skipping breakfast, but it's really hard for anyone that's used to packing a ton of calories into their morning for quick energy. It might take the full two-weeks to feel normal amounts of energy, although you'll typically feel a loss during the last hour before the eating window.

Back Off if it Seems too Problematic or Difficult

If you become emotionally upset or it becomes too much, or you begin to experience any unusual symptoms, discontinue the fast and consider dropping back or modifying the plan. Take time to analyze the situation when you can think clearly. It's possible to have a bad day and you can retry on your next fast day.

You can always modify the plan to be low-calorie during the fast instead of no-calorie. You also have the option of drinking a cup of broth during missed snack or mealtimes. It can help alleviate feelings of hunger and deprivation. Fasting should never feel like torture. If it gets too difficult, switch back to the lower fasting plan and create a new strategy.

Rethinking Your Plan

It's time to rethink the plan you picked if you feel it was a complete failure. It happens sometimes if you pick a plan that is more rigorous and demanding than the first one. One might sound easy enough, but it seems incredibly hard once you get going. A great example is to step up from the 12:12 plan to the eat-skip-eat plan. You are literally doubling your fasting time, even though you get complete days of regular meals between.

Avoid stepping up too quickly or you will become frustrated and give up. You can also experience unpleasant side effects that weren't expected, such as serious drops in blood sugar or hormonal imbalance. A sudden switch of moods can be a sign that your hormones aren't taking the drastic change that well. Feeling a little cranky is one thing, but wanting to throw objects across the room is another. Choose a plan that is not much different than the one you are on already.

Reaching the Top of Your Personal Pyramid – Enjoy the View

Setting personal goals of weight loss or improved health are all good reasons to begin an IF plan, but you will end up finding a plan that is suited so well to your lifestyle and gives you such amazing results that you'll make it a lifestyle change. It's considered the top of your pyramid and feels great to achieve. The daily routine no longer feels like a chore and seems to come more naturally. The periods without food are comfortable or only marginally challenging.

IF Plan and Leveling Up

You'll need to revisit the section about moving to a new IF plan in the previous chapter as often as necessary to move to another plan with effectiveness. Take every precaution to try and ensure it's a plan you can do and are prepared to tackle. You might find that another plan is better suited to your needs and goals than the one you are currently using.

Once you've experienced fasting, it might seem less intimidating to try a 24-hour fasting plan. You can always start with two-weeks of the Warrior Diet. It gives you a strong experience of 20 hours in fasting and 4 hours of eating window. It's a natural progression from the 16:8 and perfect for those that are used to squeezing in one meal a day on a busy schedule. The real challenge is in not snacking during the 20-hour fast.

Should it Always Be a Struggle?

If you are really struggling with your IF plan, you are aiming too high for your current abilities. The constant struggle will make you unhappy and might lead you to turn away from the benefits of IF completely. Stay within a plan and range that offers a little challenge, without seeming like a nightmare test of your food derivation withstanding abilities. Here are a few ways you can make the IF plan less of a struggle when having difficulties:

- Exit the fast and re-evaluate your plan.
- Reduce your fasting day by one until you feel better and able to keep up.
- Reduce the fasting time.
- Allow low-calorie items.
- Stop fasting temporarily and evaluate diet/nutrition intake.

Some IF plans work against the schedule you keep, lifestyle, or cause too much upheaval within your body. Remember, women are designed to have a more sensitive system when it comes to blood sugar fluctuations and hormonal imbalances. It's better to keep trying until you find the right combination that can be customized to your wants and needs.

Finding an IF Comfort Zone

Finding an IF plan that is comfortable is more than picking the one and giving it a try. It takes careful consideration and a little work from outside the plan to make it a smooth fit. Getting yourself mentally and physically prepared for fasting, on the road to a healthier diet, and developing better eating habits all work in unison to make the plan comfortable. Optimizing your start dates, end dates, and times are other specifics that can make big differences in how you feel and succeed. You are on the right track with an IF plan when:

- The start of your fast seems like a natural part of your day.

- You are able to complete your fast with little or no discomfort.
- Your energy levels feel steady and plentiful, even during the fast.
- The fasting presents little challenge until the end.
- Your focus has drifted away from food.
- You feel no urgency to overeat or binge after the fast.

Continue working with IF plans until you reach your goals with a program that doesn't continually test you. Feeling comfortable should come with a reasonable challenge, but not as a daily trial. An IF plan is there that, when adjusted the right way and prepared for properly, is one that exactly fits your wants and needs. You'll wonder why you never tried IF before.

Making the Lifestyle Switch – Enjoying the View from the Top

Give each IF plan you start a two-week trial before making the decision to switch unless you are experiencing health problems or have chosen one that's too advanced. Once you have leveled up to a point that seems comfortable for your schedule and gives you the results you want, make it your new lifestyle. You've officially reached your personal pyramid summit and can take time to enjoy the view!

DISCLAIMER

This book and the information contained inside are not to be construed or used as a replacement for sound medical advice from your primary medical practitioner. Every effort has been made to research the information thoroughly to offer sound, accurate information, but it should not serve as a replacement for medical advice from a doctor that knows your exact medical information. You should always consult with your doctor before drastically changing your diet to keep from experiencing avoidable complications and reduce risks to your health.

Your experience of any IF plan must be tempered with an understanding and awareness of possible problem signs that indicate you should stop immediately. It might require making some changes to another, gentler plan, or modifications on fasting. Do not ignore the signals and signs your body gives. To do so can lead to further health complications.

Sleeping Problems

Difficulty sleeping can come from many areas. It might be in response to other symptoms when hormones begin to fall out of balance. It can also result from your focus on food and hunger pangs. Consistent loss of sleep can lead to problems with your energy levels, mood stability, and immune system function. Chronic lack of sleep can make your life miserable at work and in your personal life.

Unexpected and Excessive Hair Loss

The head of every woman replaces strands of hair on a daily basis. The loss of a few strands in the hairbrush each morning is rarely a concern. Finding more and more hair falling out when IF fasting can be a sign that your hormones are getting out of balance or you are fatiguing your adrenal system. Discontinue the IF plan and see your doctor. It's a problem more common to women with thyroid issues, PCOS, or approaching menopause. Have your physician make the determination if fasting is the right program for you. A modified plan might be the solution.

Extreme and Non-Stop Headaches

Chronic headaches can come from many sources. Eating too many carbs and sugars on your resting days and in the eat windows can lead to what many term "hungry headaches." Headaches can also come from dehydration and not drinking enough water. The headaches can make your life miserable. It's best to stop your fast and carefully handle your nutritional and hydration needs. Avoid taking any type of pain reliever while in the fasting state. It can cause stomach upset or pain. Aspirin and other NSAIDs can cause stomach bleeding when taken without food.

Daytime Energy Drain

Experiencing low energy levels for your first week of longer fasting is normal. You'll feel drained and famished right before the fast ends. Your energy levels should return to normal or be improved as your body adapts to burning fat reserves for fuel. A lack of energy can be due to not getting the right amount of sleep, a lack of nutrition, or adrenal fatigue. You should seek the advice of your doctor before continuing with an IF plan. Specific dietary changes might be needed to feel better and set your system right for successful fasting.

Extreme Weight Loss/Gain

You should see a steady loss of fat reserves as you fast, but it shouldn't be a remarkable amount in a short period of time. Your weight loss will be permanent and gradual. Gaining weight is something that shouldn't happen unless you begin to binge-eat after your fasts. Extreme fluctuations in weight, either up or down, can be a sign of a developing eating disorder or a thyroid problem. You should discontinue fasting plans if you are experiencing eating disorders. See your doctor if you feel there may be a problem with your thyroid glands. Finding problems early allows for better results in solutions.

Mood Swings

It's not unusual to feel a little grumpy during your fast when the hours are drawing out and you want something to eat. Experiencing severe swings in mood both on and off the fast is a sign that you might be having hormonal imbalance issues. Any woman that is approaching the age of pre-menopause can easily throw hormones out of balance through drastic dietary changes. You need to back off and discontinue the fast. Begin again, slower, once your hormones seem to level out. It may be necessary to stay on a lighter IF plan to avoid future problems.

Menstrual Fluctuations

It might seem nice to have your period go away when on an IF plan, but it can be a warning sign that something is going on with your hormones. Wildly fluctuating periods can indicate that the hormones are in a state of imbalance and it can set you into premature menopause. It can also mess with fertility by interrupting normal ovulation. You should end your fasting and see your doctor. No matter how much of a relief it might seem at the time to not have a period, the long-term effects of early-onset menopause can be extreme. Find out what it will take to set your system back to normal.

Internal Body Temperature Problems

A sure sign of pre and actual menopause is a range of internal temperature fluctuations that cause hot flashes or night sweats. It's due to the variation and imbalance of hormones in the body. Exit the fasting and focus on your nutrition for a while. Try it again at a slower pace when the hormones come into balance. If you continue to experience temperature fluctuations, try a modified or extremely simple plan. Don't try to tough it out and put up with these problems. It is a sign that your hormones are in imbalance.

Dizziness or Mental Confusion

Do you feel dizzy when standing up during your fast? Do you feel dizzy or disoriented at any point? Some dizziness is expected if you are new to fasting and have begun a full day fast. You may not have eaten enough nutrients in your resting period or eating window. Mental confusion or disorientation can be a sign of other medical issues. Discontinue fasting and see your doctor right away. You might have a blood pressure problem, blood sugar, or other heart-related problem. It's best to be safe and get the clearance of your doctor before trying again.

Chapter 6: Intermittent Fasting and the Ketogenic Diet

Intermittent fasting and a ketogenic diet use different approaches to achieve the same goal. The similarities of reducing carbs, sugars, and increasing the eating of healthy fats promote adaptation of the body to burning fat as a primary source of energy. Can you safely use IF and keto diets together? This chapter explores the similarities and differences of IF and keto and how combining the two can increase your fat burning potential.

Should I Eat Carbs

The reduction of carbs is a must for both IF and the ketogenic diet, which makes it essential to understand why it's necessary to get expected results in weight loss. Knowing why high levels of carbs are a bad thing for any diet will make it easier to understand what is going on internally when you practice IF or keto dieting. Keeping track of your daily carb percentage is as important, if not more, than calories consumed.

Carbs and Carb Breakdown

Carbs like bread, rice, beans, and most types of fruit easily break down into a fuel the body can burn for energy. Carbs can be found in all processed foods and many natural sources. A high intake of 30 percent and more of your daily calories as carbs can lead to weight gain and high levels of blood sugar when activity levels are moderate or low. It's not considered healthy to maintain a higher carb intake than what your body needs on a daily basis.

What happens to excess amounts of carbs? The body will bundle them up and store them as fat deposits. The more extra carbs your diet brings into the body, the higher your weight will climb. It's the reason many people can't understand why they gain weight when they avoid sweets and drink diet beverages. The culprit could be too many carbohydrates with too little physical activity.

Reaching Ketosis

What is ketosis? Ketosis is a state the body reaches in which the level of carbs drops to the point the brain is deprived of glucose. It triggers the liver to produce ketones that can be burned for fuel to supply the brain and body with necessary energy. It's a specific interaction and triggering mechanism that cannot be reproduced by taking pills and potions. It's reached by simply removing or limiting other sources of fuel from the body.

Being in a state of ketosis is a time that produces the greatest results in losing fat build-up, especially stubborn belly fat. It's the desired state that has had nutritionists and fitness experts on the hunt for the best way to achieve this state. One is by undergoing periods of zero calorie intake, which intermittent fasting provides and the other is through the ketogenic diet. Both are viable triggers of the ketosis state.

Benefits of Ketosis

One of the biggest benefits of ketosis is the speed at which you can begin dropping weight. It begins to assist in removing fat that has been stored for months or even years. Ketosis also helps your exiting muscles become leaner. It's why getting in the state of ketosis is so desired by those trying to drop large amounts of weight and amateur or professional athletes trying to lean-out and gain muscles.

Ketosis also provides an appreciable drop in blood sugar levels. It can prove beneficial for those that are type 2 diabetic or at risk of developing diabetes. It also provides autophagy processes that conduct deep cellular cleansing of toxins from the body. It removes the clutter of dead cells and defective cell parts, pathogenic materials, and other things that lead to illness or reduced cellular function. It brings back youthful energy and action to every cell in your body.

Eliminating Empty Carbs

Not all carbs are bad for you. You should never completely drop them from your diet. You have to weigh each on a scale of importance and decide which ones are beneficial and which are empty. Empty carbs are ones like those found in sugary baked goods and candies. The carbs in fruits and vegetables can be beneficial for the antioxidants, fiber, and vitamins. The carbs in beans aren't always bad due to the fiber and protein content.

Both IF and the ketogenic diet will require that you sift through your dietary choices and give any empty carbs the axe. The rest of the carbs should be kept in balance and no more than 5 or 10 percent of your calories each day. Anything higher and you leave the state of ketosis and are once again running on the carbs you eat. Keep carbs ultra-low when fasting or doing the keto diet.

Finding Hidden Carbs

Eating foods blindly is one way to guarantee you exit ketosis on a regular basis. Foods that are packaged often hold levels of carbs that are astounding when looking at the nutrition label. You might think yogurt is healthy, which it is for the most part, but it contains a high level of carbs. It can be as much as 20 percent of your daily intake. Going much over this by adding fruit will take you out of ketosis.

The best way to avoid hidden carbs is to eat as much fresh stuff as possible and cook your own food. You can choose low-carb vegetables like bell peppers instead of white potatoes. All of your green leafy vegetables are perfect for both keto dieting and IF. The more you understand about carbs and how to keep them limited, the more successful both ketogenic diets and IF works.

Comparing IF and Keto

The comparisons of IF and keto diets show some remarkable similarities in abilities and body responses, but enough differences to warrant a closer look. No matter how similar they appear, they are in no way the same in final results and the process required to achieve them. The following are a few of the basic similarities and differences.

Both Keto and IF Improve Memory Function and Reduce Mental Fog

The ketones produced by the liver to feed the brain during a state of ketosis provide better protection and antioxidant value than spent carbs ever could. The autophagy cleansing helps clear up brain fog and increases the neurotransmitter activity, which leads to improved memory and brain function. Both ketogenic dieting and fasting are shown to give positive results, although IF has a slight advantage in being able to perform a deeper cleansing in a short amount of time. Ketogenic diets allow for cleansing on a regular basis throughout the day and night.

Keto Offers Ketosis Benefits While Feeling Full and Satisfied Nutritionally

One of the biggest differences in IF and keto dieting is that one requires an uncomfortable period of taking in no calories. The other gives you the ketosis state benefits while filling up on nutritious, satisfying foods. IF can seem a bit like food deprivation until your system gets adjusted to the fasting periods. Some plans require a complete 24-hour fast, whereas others allow small windows of opportunity to eat. The keto diet is a standard daily routine. What you might find lacking in keto dieting is variety, unless you become nutritionally aware of all the items you can eat without restriction.

IF Gives a Deeper Autophagy Response

Completely fasting from food and calories for up to a day at a time triggers a deeper round of autophagy response than the standard keto dieting. Every round of fasting you do will initiate the same response to a deeper level, giving your body a needed detox and boost in health. The benefits of deep autophagy begin to fall after the 48-hour mark, which is well beyond most IF fasting periods.

Both Keto and IF Provide Ketosis Fat Burning Advantages

The ability to enter into the state of ketosis is what provides the all-important fat burning capabilities that go beyond anything that calorie restriction can do. Both keto diets and IF give you the advantage in fat burning that happens without any special efforts or work other than following your specified plans and food list. Standard dieting involves extensive calorie counting and can lead to frustration in feeling deprived. The keto diet gives plenty of options that allow you to feel full and IF gives you open eating windows with very few restrictions, other than carbs.

The Keto Diet Puts You in Ketosis State for Long Periods of Time

A ketogenic diet places your body in a ketosis state for as long as it is you are reducing carbs to a level that fat burning is necessary. Your body turns into a literal fat burning machine day and night. The only times this process stops are when the carb total is more than what your body needs to operate. Your liver will then stop providing ketones and the carbs will be burned for fuel. IF only provides the fat burning during the fast. The body will leave ketosis state once the eating window starts and you eat regular foods.

IF Fasting Can Be Frustrating Under Stress

Fasting is something that your body can become accustomed to, but there are times that everything seems to be going wrong and it becomes a source of frustration. It's difficult to do a lot of strenuous activities when you are in the middle of a longer fast. You have energy, but extensive activities like moving furniture can be trying. The keto diet keeps you in constant supply of the needed nutrients to stay active all day, in all activities.

Keto Diets Can Be Hard to Maintain Long-Term

Harvard Medical School has made numerous attempts over the years to stay in contact with those they have studied using the ketogenic diet. Most have reported falling off the diet plan after a year or two citing a variety of reasons it was difficult to continue using the keto plan. Most find that the fat burning slows after a few months, but this is due to the extraordinary amount of fat burning that has already taken place. The failure to stay on the diet is more likely due to reaching personal weight loss and muscle leaning goals.

IF and Keto – An Auspicious Marriage

Specific good things happen when pairing IF and the ketogenic diet. It's a sensible way to get continuous benefits similar to doing one or the other alone. It can enhance the benefits of one or the other in certain aspects.

IF Makes Switching to a Keto Diet More Comfortable

Taking on the keto diet from standard diets can be more than a little uncomfortable. It can cause a sluggish flu-like feeling for a few days. It's termed "keto flu." Starting with an IF plan that has at least a 12-hour fast period can eliminate or reduce these symptoms. You will already have your body moving towards ketosis and becoming fat adapted.

Using an IF plan before starting the keto diet will allow you to enter ketosis sooner than using the keto diet alone. It leads to a better feeling of comfortable weight loss, dieting, and fasting. Everything meshes together at a quicker pace. The keto diet is filled with all of the foods you need to succeed with IF. You won't feel yourself slipping gears and having the diet clash with the fasting.

IF and Keto Diet Together Allow for Less Hormone Fluctuation

Hormonal imbalance is an important factor for women to keep in mind and monitor. It can happen quickly and be hard to get back under control. The biggest risk for hormonal imbalance is with women that already experience an imbalance or are close to and entering menopause. The slightest dietary changes are often all it takes to send things wildly out of control. You can feel fine one day and be an emotional wreck the next.

The ketogenic diet and IF complement one another by their being less variances in carbs. The keto diet is slim on carbs, which produces less insulin response. It's the switching from glycogen to insulin that brings about the ups and downs of hormonal imbalance. The blood sugar levels will never spike if you truly follow the IF plan and keto diet for the eating windows.

Better Stable Energy with Ketosis-Friendly Foods

Attempting to do the IF plan of your choice can result in problems if your diet remains unhealthy. Loading it with foods that are high in carbs means your body will blow through the fuel and you'll be left feeling empty. The body will have to switch channels and begin burning fat instead. It's your ultimate goal, but it's easier to already be in the flow of fat burning when you fast.

You'll avoid that lurch in your system that is required when changing gears to fat burning from carb burning. The energy you have at the start will continue unabated. Your body will stay focused on staying in operation using ketones. The typical drag you feel as you near the end of a longer fast will disappear. It becomes a simple process to move through the fats and on into your eating window. The focus on food completely goes away.

Continual Fat Loss

You already know that the fasting with IF begins a fast-pace of burning fat as there is no other fuel available when your intake of calories is zero. Without the keto diet, the fat burning would end until the next fast window begins. Extend your fat burning by using the keto diet during the eating windows.

Autophagy will be continual, even if it's to a lesser degree.

Using one or the other will provide a level of fat burning that's not available with most other diet methods. It's the combination that can maximize your fat burning and weight loss potential with both IF and the keto diet. Why not get the most from your efforts and time spent fasting and dieting? Add in some exercise and you have the perfect fat trimming plan.

Complete Self-Healing

Combining the ketogenic diet and IF is one way to ensure you are getting the most complete self-healing that's available to you through the natural autophagy process. The IF fasting will trigger the autophagy sooner than it would with the keto only dieting. Every cell in your body will benefit greatly from removing the cellular "trash" that gets left behind as cells are regenerated over time.

The keto dieting will provide the long-term self-healing that autophagy offers. You will benefit from continual, round-the-clock cellular cleansing and repair that can turn back the hands of time on your body. The results are better overall health and a feeling of well-being.

Benefits

Choosing to combine an IF plan with the ketogenic diet will offer you increased benefits that can help you reach your goals faster. It's also a way to reach your goals in a more comfortable and manageable way. Imagine being able to melt away stubborn body fat without a huge struggle. The right IF plan coupled with the keto diet can make it the smoothest weight loss experience you've ever tried.

Stabilized Hormone Levels

Keeping the hormones from getting out of sorts is one of the most important things for any woman trying to lose weight through dietary methods. Use the combination of IF and the keto diet to give your body the opportunity to easily stay in a healthy hormonal balance. You'll have a more pleasant experience in burning away the pounds.

Stabilized Blood Sugar Levels

Get off the blood sugar roller coaster by benefitting from the low-carb keto diet. Avoid uncomfortable and dangerous spikes in blood sugar levels that switching from a normal carb intake to fasting can bring. You'll be far less likely to experience any moments of weakness or dizziness during fasting. Your fasting time will pass by without notice, especially when staying busy. The ability to safeguard yourself against diabetes by reducing blood sugar is priceless.

Enduring Energy Source

Enjoy an almost endless source of energy when fasting and gaining your nutrition from a ketogenic diet. You will feel fuller as you enter your fast and not feel completely drained of nutrition from the start. Your body will be filled with an abundant source of healthy fats, lean protein, and the right amount of carbs to keep ketosis moving forward.

Complementary Diet to Fasting

The healthy proteins that are grass-fed, avocados, eggs, green leafy vegetables, peppers, sweet potatoes, and anti-oxidant rich fruits of a keto diet will all help fuel you to and through a more successful fast. No other diet out there works in tandem to provide stronger results than the combination of ketogenic dieting and IF. The parallel demands and outcomes make them the perfect to work together for increased fat burning and health improvement.

Maximum Fat Burning Plan

Most diets work by restricting calories and making it impossible for the body to burn any more than what you give. The ketogenic diet and IF plans are designed to use your own natural ability to burn fat to your advantage. You can get a jumpstart on results and begin losing steady amounts of fat, resulting in permanent weight loss right away. You'll lose pounds of fat your first week and the fat burning will continue as long as you keep your body in the ketosis state.

Easier Transition to Fat Adaption

Your body is said to be fat adapted once it begins the regular process of burning the fats for energy production. The quickest way to get your body doing this is through longer fasting. Use of the 16:8 IF plan and following with the keto diet ensures the body keeps burning fat for fuel at a regular pace until reaching your desired weight loss goal.

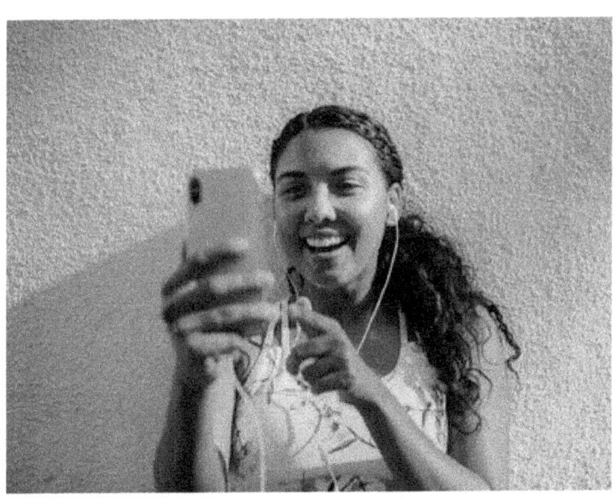

Feel Younger and Healthier

Not only does consistent detoxification of your body and maintaining cellular performance a way to physically feel better each day, it also brings back the energy levels you enjoyed years ago. It's a natural way to defeat the aging process and works better than any chemical product ever could. Your own body functions can do more to promote natural healing and cleansing than anything a pharmacist or pharmaceutical company can invent.

Chapter 7: Useful Techniques and Other IF Hacks

Getting started and maintaining an IF plan is made easier using the special techniques and hacks presented in this chapter. Learn the easiest ways to track your calories, reduce your carbs, find sources of healthy fats, and how to tell if you're really hungry. Arm yourself with the knowledge you need to develop a winning strategy.

Calorie Tracking Made Easy

You will have times that counting calories are essential. When using a modified fast with restricted amounts of calorie intake, counting is necessary. It doesn't have to be a hassle. The following are a few sensible solutions to making calorie counting possible without taking up too much of your time.

Plan Your Calories in Advance

Plan the foods you'll eat in your fasting periods in advance and have the calories already calculated. Keep lists easy to find that have the calorie values for single servings of the meats you use and the basic vegetables. The inside doors of your cupboards are handy places to place them where they are out of the way. Check the labels of any packaged or canned foods. It should have the serving size and calories per serving listed. You can easily mark this down and track everything you eat during your restricted timeframe.

Journal the Foods Eaten, Times, and Other Important Data

Keep your journal handy to mark down any foods you eat, times, amount, and any other data you need to track. It's helpful if you are entering a restricted calorie portion without having anything planned or you are away from home.

Use an App like MyFitnessPal

Apps are available like MyFitnessPal that can help you count calories and track what you eat and when. It makes it easier than ever before. Most fitness apps have a calorie tracking feature. Find one to use that is easy and uncomplicated.

Don't Count Every Calorie Beyond Calorie Restricted Times

Make it easier on yourself and avoid counting calories when you don't have to. Write down the foods you eat on resting days and eating windows to monitor that you're getting enough nutrition and aren't binging on food. It can help pinpoint any flaws in your eating that could be leading you down a path that can derail your goals. Make it easy to get back on track by monitoring eating habits.

Stick with What You Know is Low Calorie

Eating out is easy with an IF plan but stick with things you know contain low-calorie ingredients. Don't go for exotic mixtures that are impossible to know the calorie count. It's the best way to avoid throwing yourself overboard and overeating.

Reduced Carb Intake

It can't be overstated how important your reduction in carbs in your diet will help in success with the IF plans. Although going completely carb-free is virtually impossible, you can reduce them to a level that your entire IF experience is pleasant, with fewer problematic symptoms.

Why Reduce Carbs?

One of the biggest reasons to reduce carbs is that it translates to sugar in your body. It defeats the purpose of an IF plan. Your goal is to hit ketosis state and begin burning fat. Your body will not do this if there is a ready-source of easy to burn fuel like carbs. Think about this the next time you feel tempted to make some toast or eat a bagel.

Carbs and Cravings

A steady diet of carbs keeps those hungry hormones rooting around for something more. You will have more cravings and feelings of food deprivation if you keep your main diet loaded with carbohydrates and sugars. Begin to reduce the amounts as you near your start date of the IF plan.

Increase Feelings of Fullness and Food Satisfaction

Low-carb foods are known to give you a fuller sensation for a longer period of time. When you are full and stay full, your hunger is satisfied. Your attention span will turn to other things beyond food. Never feeling hunger satiation means you'll struggle with every fast. Your blood sugar will fluctuate and experiences of weakness or dizziness can appear. The seeming lack of food will have you eating everything under the sun when eating windows open. A low-carb diet will ensure you have less hunger pangs, doubts about the plan, and you'll stick to the fast out to the end.

Great Low-Carb Foods

Here is a list of low carb meats that are great to create a healthy eating routine with:

- Grass-fed beef
- Chicken
- Shrimp
- Trout
- Haddock
- Bacon
- Salmon
- Sardines
- Tuna
- Turkey
- Veal
- Cod
- Catfish
- Venison
- Jerky
- Shellfish

- Mackerel

Here is a list of low-carb vegetables:

- Cabbage
- Tomatoes
- Zucchini
- Onions
- Shallots
- Kale
- Broccoli
- Asparagus
- Green beans
- Cauliflower
- Brussels Sprouts
- Eggplant
- Cucumber
- Bell Peppers
- Mushrooms
- Swiss chard
- Spinach
- Collard greens
- Mustard greens

Here are a few low-carb fruits:

- Strawberries
- Blueberries
- Apricots
- Avocado
- Olives
- Grapefruit
- Lemon
- Oranges
- Kiwis

Low-carb seeds and nuts:

- Almonds
- Walnuts
- Hazelnuts
- Chia seeds
- Pumpkin seeds
- Sunflower seeds
- Macadamia nuts
- Peanuts
- Cashews
- Flax seeds

Low-carb dairy:

- Cheese
- Greek yogurt
- Heavy cream

You can select from a world of spices that help give each dish you make an original flavor. More flavor-infused foods will also help satisfy hunger. Low-carb choices give you a great selection to work with to make healthy meals that leave you feeling full.

Healthy Fat

Fat has been looked at the enemy for decades when it comes to eating healthy and attempting to lose weight. Modern research methods have revealed that some high-fat foods are actually great for you and contain more than fat. Many are loaded with vitamins and minerals, antioxidants, and protein. The benefits, when introduced in the IF plan diet, are undeniable.

Why You Need Healthy Fats for the IF Plan

Introducing fats to your body through diet is an easy way to train it to begin using it for fuel. Lower the carbs and increase the healthy fats and the body will quickly make the switch. Although they have discovered that a certain amount of fat is healthy, they can't be just any fats. Some fats can contribute to heart and cardiovascular disease. The healthier varieties offer more than fat and often give you a good source of protein, which you need for weight loss.

Creating a Steady Energy Source

Including healthy fats in your diet give a non-stop source of fuel for your body, which means you won't experience any of the possible drains that happen with eating windows filled with processed, sugary, and high-carb foods. As the food you consume is burned during your fast, the body switches over and begins using the stored fat, producing weight loss. It's a smooth transition that makes the fast one that allows for plenty of energy to get things done.

Moving Away from the Carbs and Sugars to the Healthy Fat Sources

The meals you make should always contain a selection of leafy greens for the fiber and ability to make you feel full. It also provides a great source of vitamins. Trade unhealthy cuts of meat and processed meats out of your diet and switch to healthy fat varieties, such as grass-fed beef and seafood. You should only eat whole grains, whole-wheat pasta, and brown rice in moderation. You can quickly end up in carb overload. Try honey as a sweetener over sugar. Try a sliced cucumber and wedge of cheese for a snack instead of a piece of cake.

Healthy Fat Choice

Are you mystified at what the choices are for healthy fats? It's understandable since most health classes and instructions on nutrition have veered people away from fats for so long. Here are a few items you can add to your arsenal that are high in healthy fats and other nutritional goodies:

- Eggs
- Cheese
- Nuts
- Lean, grass-fed beef
- Fatty fish
- Chia seeds
- Dark chocolate
- Avocados
- Yogurt
- Cottage cheese
- Olive oil
- Avocado oil

Sugar and Starch

Sugar is considered a carbohydrate and starch, a complex carbohydrate. Both will eventually be broken down and create a quick rise in insulin response. Your blood sugar level is nearly immediately impacted. Your body will burn sugar first and then work on the starches well before consideration of burning stored fats.

Why Set Limits on Sugar?

You must reign in your dietary intake of sugar if you want to lose weight using IF or avoid uncomfortable spikes in blood sugar. The amounts of items that can contain sugar are astounding. Eating a piece of fried chicken can cause your blood sugar to rise due to the flour breading. Here are a few items to avoid:

- Flour and cornmeal
- Tortillas and bread
- Cookies, cakes, and other baked goods
- Sweetened cereal
- Dried and canned fruit
- Canned or bottled spaghetti sauce
- Condiments and salad dressing
- Sweetened beverages, including vitamin water and sports drinks
- Non-organic honey and syrups

How to Avoid Sugar in the Diet

- Grill meats or sauté using virgin olive oil instead of breading and frying.

- Sweeten drinks or foods with organic honey.
- Eat fresh fruits in limited quantities to satisfy sweet tooth.
- Eliminate flour and flour-containing products from your diet and only add as you need.
- Avoid sugar-free items as it still contains sugar alcohol, which can be just as trying on your body.
- Switch to filling proteins, like eggs in the morning instead of sugary cereals and drinks.

Why Set Limits on Starch?

Starch, as a complex carbohydrate, is another way to wreck your IF progress if you aren't careful. It also breaks down into a readily available fuel and your body will quickly put it into the system, raising blood sugar levels. A few examples of foods with high levels of starch are:

- Cereal
- Oats

- Potatoes, although still recommended for diet due to other nutrition
- Corn, although still recommended for fiber and nutrients
- Pasta
- Rice
- Bread
- Instant noodles
- Flour
- Crackers
- Pretzels

How to Avoid Starch in the Diet

- Choose fresh fruit and vegetable snacks like cucumber slices, apple slices, and top with thinly sliced cheese.
- Switch to broiled and stir-fry vegetables as sides and put away the rice and pasta.
- Check the ingredients list of packaged foods to see if there are any starch-laden items.
- Avoid purchasing "quick-fix" or "instant" food items. Either the starches or preservatives will get you.

- Use corn and potatoes sparingly unless you are doing regular exercise routines. These are a good source of carbs for the ultra-active individual.
- Only eat bread-related items as whole grain, sparingly. Kick flour to the curb.

Knowing you have the backup of beverages to help fill an empty void, keep you hydrated, and get you through to the eating window will help you enter comfortably into a fast. You must decide before starting if you will allow any sort of added calories. Adding a splash of creamer to coffee or tea will add a few calories, although not enough to bring you out of ketosis.

Water

Water will be your biggest source of hydration during your fast. Make sure you increase your normal intake by as many as 5 or 6 glasses due to no food. Your body normally extracts water from all the food eaten.

Unsweetened Coffee and Black Tea

Unsweetened coffee and black tea will be your go-to drink when you are feeling weakened and hungry. Both tea and coffee contain caffeine, which has a certain level of hunger suppression qualities. Be sparing with the creamer if you plan to drink numerous cups. Switch to decaf and try drinking it black. If it bothers your stomach, move on to something else. You don't want a stomach ache from coffee or tea on top of hunger pangs.

Green Tea

Green tea is another great beverage for hydration and adds antioxidants to the mix. It's good served both hot or cold. You can also look into a variety of different herbal teas and mixes. The herbs add zero calories to the water, but the flavor might be something that alleviates hunger and distracts you from the fast.

Ginger Tea

Ginger tea is great because it tastes almost like a soup. Add a teaspoon to hot water, stir, and sip when cool enough to do so. You can add a dash of salt and pepper to really bring the flavor home. Ginger is filled with antibiotic qualities for healing and immune system support. It remains a drink with no calories with added spices.

Clear Broth

Broth made from bone marrow or vegetables is a way to kill serious hunger pangs without adding a ton of calories. It's the perfect beverage for those on a modified diet or if you are afraid of completely falling off your fast. It can also be a way to keep your sodium levels up for workouts but should be avoided if you have high blood pressure or heart disease.

Fruit Infused Water or Seltzer Water

Add a few blueberries, strawberry, raspberries, or an orange slice to your water or seltzer water and let it sit in the fridge. The flavor of the fruit will intermingle with the water and you'll have an all-natural fruit flavored drink.

Many people are scared to try fasting due to the belief they will be completely consumed with thoughts of food and terrible hunger pangs. It's true that you will be somewhat food-focused in the beginning and will feel a few hunger pangs, the truth is the feeling of hunger will subside. As you break the food habits and mental conditioning of a three-meal-a-day system, the fasts become easier to get through.

Eating as a Behavior Rather than a Need

Much like Pavlov's dog in studies where ringing the bell became associated with food, humans tend to start salivating and feeling hunger pangs with specific associated stimuli. Looking at the clock and realizing it's a standard mealtime can be all it takes to get your tummy going. Fasting is a great way to disconnect from those stimuli and reset your hunger needs and triggers.

Conditioned Hunger Response

A conditioned response to hunger is one where you are seeing a visual representation of people eating in magazines, movies, or on television. You may have been perfectly fine until seeing that taco commercial or looking at an advertisement for a steakhouse. All of a sudden, your stomach starts grumbling and you can't get your mind off food. Staying busy and not dwelling on it is about the best cure when a commercial or ad has captured your attention.

Unconditioned Hunger Response

Unconditioned response to hunger is what comes to us through our senses. If you see or smell food, you might begin to have a hunger response in your body. It's one reason that hanging out with friends or family at a restaurant or barbecue can be difficult if you are on a fast. It takes a ton of willpower to overcome the natural unconditioned response to want to eat when food is present.

It's easier to try and set your fasting days where they don't conflict with prearranged plans. Don't go into a situation thinking you are superhuman. Anyone can fall with the right temptation and your aunt's cheesecake might be just the thing you can't resist!

Eat When You Need to Eat

Breaking the chains of behavioral eating patterns and addictions is the best way to get to a healthy weight and maintain. Fasting with IF is one way to do this painlessly and in a way that's safe. Your body will learn to only send you cues to eat when it needs food. You might not even get signals to eat. Hunger pangs tend to diminish. Never skip an eating window without intending to extend your fasting. You can set your system out of whack.

Some people pull back from thoughts of fasting due to irrational fears of starvation. The fasting involved with IF plans will not take you anywhere near the threshold of complete starvation. It's actually proven to be beneficial to your health and can extend your lifespan by ridding the body of toxins.

How Long Can a Person Last Without Food?

No real studies exist that follow a person from ceasing to take in nourishment to the time of death, but a few cases have been noted and logged. Hunger strikes in the UK decades ago had one hunger strike victim lasting 40 days and another 73 days. Both were allowed water and did virtually nothing but lie in a cot until death. You have a far less chance of surviving more than 3 weeks if you are up and active.

It's All About BMI

A supermodel has an average BMI or body mass index of 17. The average woman has a

BMI of 18.5-24. If a woman of 5-feet, 7-inches, weighing 145 pounds, and consuming a daily diet of 2,400 calories quits eating, she will live about 3-weeks. It is less time if she no longer drinks water as well. During the process of complete starvation, the body consumes between 25 and 50 percent of their available BMI. A woman with a high BMI could live slightly longer without food, but one of 18 BMI or lower might not make it more than 2 weeks.

Why Sensible Fasting Doesn't Lead to Starvation

Hunger pangs with sensible fasting do not equate to starvation. It does show that the body has the amazing ability to create the energy needed from stored fat reserves, which gives anyone hope that has been trying to lose weight on a myriad of unsuccessful diets. Fasting for 12 hours, 16 hours, or even a week will not lead to a premature ending. It will lead to incredible amounts of deep cleansing and fat burning.

Fasting and Electrolyte Water

Taking in the vital nourishment necessary during the eating windows and staying hydrated with water and electrolyte water will keep you in great shape as you move through your IF plan. Adding dietary supplements of vitamins and minerals can also prove beneficial for those that like the longer fasting.

The next chapter will focus on a few of the common pitfalls and how to avoid them. Keep your journal handy and take notes. You want your first IF experience to be a complete success!

Chapter 8: Common Pitfalls

Avoiding some of the more common mistakes and pitfalls with IF is the best way to give yourself every chance to succeed. This chapter will help guide you away from making some of the mistakes that can make IF more complicated, ineffective, or discouraging.

Choosing the Wrong Plan

Choosing the wrong IF plan can cause you problems from the start. Too much frustration can lead to giving up on the idea of intermittent fasting altogether. Below are the most common mistakes made in choosing and how to avoid this problem.

Starting Too Ambitious

Taking on too much too soon can spell disaster with fasting. Immediately jumping into a 24-hour fast or 16:8 plan without previously experiencing a fast is an overly ambitious idea. You could end up with your blood sugar plummeting and feeling disoriented or woozy. No amount of water will make this go away. You need to end the fast and rethink your strategy.

If you have never undergone any lengthy fasting, start slower. Make sure you have taken the time to properly prepare with nutrition and hydration. 16 hours without food and conducting business as usual can be tough if you're used to three timely meals a day. 24 hours is even longer. Back the fast up to 12 hours for the first two fasting days and expand to 14 hours each the next week. If that goes well, do two weeks at 16-hour fasts.

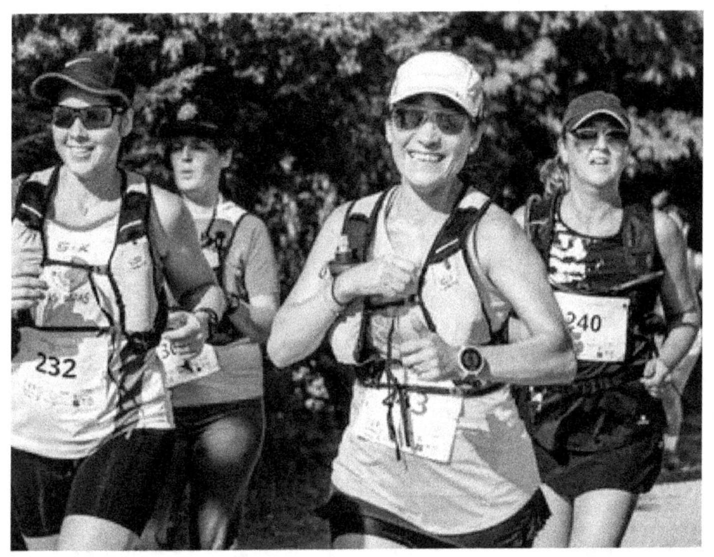

Too Much Fasting for an Active Lifestyle

Did you choose the alternate day 24-hour fasting or the Warrior Diet and find it difficult to manage with your active lifestyle? Are you lacking energy towards the end of the fast? If you are constantly on the go, do strenuous work, or daily extreme workouts, starting off with a rough 24 or 20-hour fast might not seem agreeable.

Longer fasts can be done while maintaining high levels of activity, but you should optimally have one eating window within two hours of your activity. You need to up your protein and carbs also to accommodate for extra activity. You might find it more comfortable to switch to the 16:8 fasting plan or increase your nutrition during the Warrior Diet eating window.

Wrong Plan for Desired Results

Going full tilt on a major fasting plan when all you want to do is a little light detox might be a problem. Choosing too light of a plan when you need to drop some weight might produce little results. Going far above or below your goals will also lead to frustration and wanting to give up. It doesn't hurt to choose a plan that is tougher and challenges you, as the results will be even better than desired or expected. Undershooting the goal will bring a feeling of defeat and that you've wasted your time.

Lighter detox and weight concerns can often be handled with the modified fasting or 12:12 plan. You won't have any problems handling the fasts. You'll be better encouraged to stick with it.

Maintaining nutritional balance is an important part of successful IF. Lacking the basics of what you need to comfortably roll along will set you up for a miserable experience. Too much food can set yourself up for wild drops in blood sugar. You could overshoot your calorie needs and end up never losing weight. Eating too little will leave you feeling weak and not able to complete the fast.

It might seem odd that hunger pangs go away, but it's a common experience with IF. Make sure you eat your necessary meals when the eating window opens. You need the calories, whether you feel like eating or not. Monitor that you don't overeat when off the fast, although this is a rare problem with IF. Finding the proper balance of nutrition and eating filling foods will see you through the longer fasts.

Binge Eating or Make-Up Eating

It can happen that food deprivation thoughts get stuck in your head and plunge you into an eating disorder called binge eating. As soon as the fast ends, you are grabbing everything you know you shouldn't eat. It's not a common problem, but you should monitor the amount of food you eat when off the fast. It doesn't take much to end up eating as many calories as you saved by fasting.

You can somewhat control this by limiting eating to times you are hungry or for basic nutritional need. If it continues, discontinue the fasting and try a more modified version.

What Happens When You Don't Feel Hungry?

What is happening when you come off your fast and don't feel hungry? It might seem bizarre but is a commonly noted experience amongst fasters. It's not a bad thing. The lack of hunger means the fasting is working in getting you to perfect ketosis state. Your body is sustaining itself with the reserves of fat. You are experiencing real, steady fat burning.

The only caution with this is to remind yourself that you must eat a meal before fasting again. As nice as it is to feel the steady hum of perfect ketosis, it can all go to heck by starting another fast without the nutrients you need. You'll throw everything off and feel miserable in the process.

Eat Normal Meals and Don't Skip

Unless you have chosen the random meal skipping IF plan, don't skip any of your resting days or eating window meals. It's your chance to add the nutrients and belly-filling items you need to stave off hunger pangs. You will steadily lose focus on food, but remain steadfast in making sure to intake the right calories and healthy foods.

Don't try and squeeze two big meals into a 4-hour eating window. You'll end up feeling uncomfortably full. Eat a reasonably sized meal and maybe a snack at the end. The whole idea behind IF is to lose the calories and not find ways to add them back in. You'll do better by keeping your meals at normal intervals and size. The food will digest easier and you'll have fewer problems with constipation.

Do You Drink Enough?

You will struggle with fasting if you have a habit of not drinking enough water every day. Make sure you are starting your IF plan on good footing and a picture of good health. The body is anywhere from 60-78 percent water and needs to be maintained throughout the IF process.

Starting a Fast in Dehydration Mode

Being dehydrated at the beginning of your fast might bring it to a close quicker than you want. It depends on whether you can overlook the discomfort and catch up on hydration enough within the span of time of the fast. It's hard to catch up on missed hydration moments over a few hours span. A few signs of dehydration to look for are:

- Excessively dry skin
- Always thirsty
- Low urine output
- Pains or twinges in the kidneys or lower back area
- Headaches

A lack of proper hydration makes it difficult for your body to perform many of the chemical and metabolic processes it takes to lose weight. You are defeating your purpose and goal before you even begin the first fast.

Hydration and Headaches

The headache that comes from a lack of proper hydration is one that is both prolific and memorable. It's like one of the worst migraines imaginable at times. All you can do is try and hydrate with water before it gets too bad. If it takes hold, simply end the fast and find a quiet area to nurse yourself back to health. The pain can raise your blood pressure so don't try to struggle your way through the fast. End it and try again another time.

Headaches can also be caused by a lack of proper nutrients. Either way, you need to stop the fast and take care of your nutritional or hydration needs before trying the fast again. Give it a few days. Don't try it again after drinking a couple of extra glasses of water.

Have Choices Available in Addition to Water

Are you tired of water all the time? Is your schedule too busy to stop and make specialty drinks when you're fasting? Take time beforehand to brew some tea, make up some chilled green tea, or add fruit to your filtered, chilled water. You'll feel better prepared by doing all of this ahead of time. The easier you make it seem, the more you'll want to stick with your IF plan.

Check the cupboards to ensure you have everything you need before the fast day. Coffee, tea, broths, or spices to concoct your own specialty drink will make the fast pass by in a more pleasant fashion. Often, it's reverting to the use of flavors that help curb and quell strong hunger pangs. It will help keep you moving forward towards losing weight. Keep enough variety on hand to keep your taste buds from getting bored.

Your specific dietary choices can have great bearing on whether the fasting lasts or has to be adjusted and modified. Eat as high-quality of a diet as is affordable. Strip away the empty calories and begin eating things that add real value to your body. Junk food should be a thing of the past, or at least for the most part. The healthier the foundation of diet is at the start, the easier the fast and IF plan will seem. Keep cognizant of your nutritional choices, whether you have an active IF plan going or not. Do it for a healthier body at any time.

Have You Ditched Most of the Carbs?

Carbs might seem like no big deal, but they become a big deal in the middle of your fast. Too many can have your blood sugar all over the map and throw your hormones out of balance. The hormones control your level of hunger pangs, mood, and irritability levels. You can easily turn into someone that's difficult to spend time around. Carb reduction is too simple a task to let slide by unnoticed.

Be honest about your carb intake. Revisit your journal about the foods you eat to refresh your memory. You might have a bigger carb problem than you realize. You may find out that carb reduction makes you feel better all the time, especially if you are teetering on the edge of diabetes type 2.

Did You Reduce the Sugars and Starches?

Maintaining a diet high in sugars and starch content will ensure your blood sugar drops like a rock when you get rolling with the fast. Why? Your body is looking for that quick fix of fast-burning fuel that only sugars provide. Oh, it will eventually give up and start burning the fat, but you'll be might uncomfortable in the process. It's better to prepare ahead and drop the empty calories, processed junk, and high-sugar/starchy foods.

Keep the items on hand you need to answer your sweet tooth cravings after the fast. What girl doesn't enjoy chocolate? Dark chocolate in moderate amounts will hit the spot. It can keep you from grabbing a quick cookie or donut. Don't leave unhealthy snack items around the house that try your willpower. You might find that old habits die hard when new to a dietary transition.

Are You Eating Enough Greens and Healthy Fat?

The leafy greens in your diet will be what carry you through the longer fasts without feeling uncomfortable hunger pangs. Feeling full for longer time spans are the key to fasting success. You'll never feel deprived if you're incorporating enough greens. You can use them raw in salads, boiled, broiled, or steamed. It can be a base for your meats or the main part of your lunch treat.

Load up on the healthy fats before your fasting. You need to give your body the nutritional materials it needs to make the transition to ketosis state easier and faster. The better you do this step, the better the final results will be. You have the ability to maximize the benefits by making healthy choices and using good dietary judgment.

Are you excited to get started with your chosen IF plan? Take all the time you need to do the right preparations. Make a checklist to ensure you haven't forgotten any detail. Go over your chosen plan again to guarantee it's the best one for you. The right prep work is as important as diet and hydration when it comes to crossing the finish line.

Don't Start Your IF Plan Before You're Ready

You might read this book cover to cover and want to jump up and start the IF plan tomorrow. Will you really be ready tomorrow? Is everything as it should be with your diet and hydration? Do you have all of the supplies you need to make this work? Are you harboring tempting foods in your refrigerator or cupboard that can end your fast before it really starts?

The date you start isn't as important as making sure you are absolutely ready on that date. Take a couple of weeks and start a diet that will both complement and help you with the IF plan. Try a modified version of the ketogenic diet. The head start will make it much easier on your first fast.

Don't Level Up if You're Struggling Where You Are

Have you noticed a difference in how well your jeans fit? Two weeks can make a big difference, especially when you first start the IF plan. You might be anxious to push things along a little faster. Choosing a tougher level should only be done when you are totally comfortable with the one you are doing now. If you still struggle in any way with your fast – put off any changes.

Not only can make it even more difficult to struggle through a tougher and longer fast, it can discourage you and make you drop fasting altogether. It can also cause health problems by tossing your hormones into complete imbalance. Slow and easy are the best ways for women to level up in IF. The mere increase in the hormones that cause hunger can be enough to send your hormones into outer orbits. What seemed like a pleasant experience before can suddenly become nightmarish?

Don't Expand the Fasts Too Far

If one full 24-hour fast is good, maybe two are better. It's not always the case. You can expand to multiple-day fasts, but not right out of the starting gate. Give your body time to adjust to a completely new diet and routine. If you are only doing two full days of fast each week, add another day in a couple of weeks if everything is going well.

Keep looking over your journal notes and make additional adjustments as they are needed. Check with your body that it's handling everything okay. Are you experiencing any symptoms that have gone ignored? Are you steadily losing weight, but not at an alarming rate? Monitor often.

Don't Give Up Too Early

Are you in the middle of a 24-hour fast and suddenly feel overwhelmed? Are you near the end and feeling so famished and exhausted it makes you want to cry? Don't give up! You'll regret it later if it's simply a momentary weakness. Hang in there for all it's worth unless you are experiencing a health problem. The physical discomforts can be overcome. The mental and emotional battle can be won!

Are You Feeling Weak at the End?

It's not unusual to feel weakness and tiredness at the very end of your fast. You may have had incredible amounts of energy all day, but nearing the end can prove tiring. It might be the best time to grab a cup of coffee and see if it perks you up. If not, try going for a short walk in fresh air. A change of scenery or temperature can completely change your feelings of tiredness or sluggishness.

Write down how you are feeling in your journal and do some researching into whether you are getting the right amount of nutrition before you start the fast. You might have to increase your overall calories or introduce more filling foods that are slower to be digested. It might not help at the moment but can improve your experience going forward.

Try Coffee and Creamer or Broth Before Giving Up

Weakness or a loss of energy halfway through your fast is not a good thing. It means the struggle will be one that lasts for a while, if not the remainder of your fast. It's usually a sign that you aren't getting enough nutrition or you jumped the shark on IF plans without being ready. If you leveled up too quickly, it might be better to simply end the fast.

Before giving up, give a cup of black coffee or black tea a try. It might get rid of any hunger pangs. If you are merely feeling tired and sluggish, try a cup of broth. You can also add a tablespoon of creamer to your coffee and see if the few calories provided perk you up. It usually offers an immediate rise in energy levels.

Take a Few Moments to Yourself

Are you upset and feel unable to continue the fast? Distractions, stress, and emotional turmoil can interfere with fasting. Take time to separate off from others when you can and try to calm down. It might have something to do with your immediate environment. Unexpected demands at work, crying kids, burning the evening meal, or arguments with your partner can set your nerves on edge.

Take a long walk or find somewhere calm and peaceful to sit for a few moments. Collect your thoughts and breathe in the quiet. It could be a slight hormonal imbalance that causes you to feel irritable that day, but you can work through it and stay on track. Drink a glass of herbal tea and spend quality time in a peaceful room or outdoor setting.

The final chapter ahead will introduce you to some great recipes to start you on your road to ultimate health and dramatic weight loss. Are you ready to begin creating custom meals that keep the momentum of your IF plan going? Keep reading!

Chapter 9: Recipe Examples

Here are a few recipes to get you started on your healthy IF journey!

Breakfast Recipes

You can enjoy one of these tasty combinations on your resting day, or switch up some of the ingredients to something more customized to your personal preference. You can use any type of nuts and berries with your yogurt and change the meal of the scrambled egg dish to any healthy fat alternative. Add an ounce of shredded cheese and a few spinach leaves for even more protein and vitamin power.

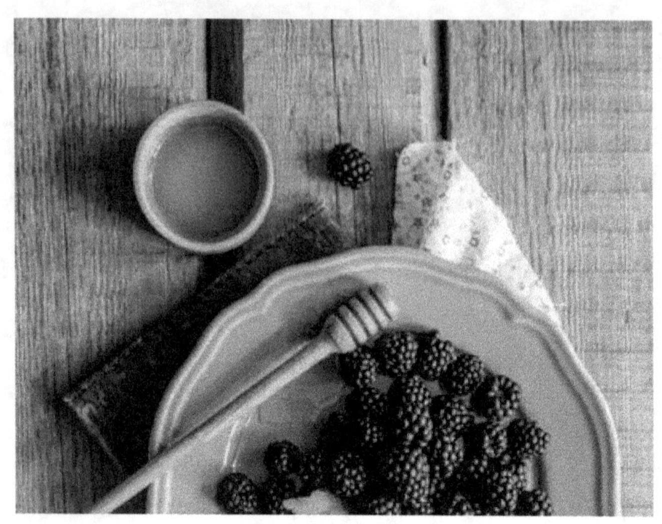

Greek Yogurt with Honey, Berries, and Nuts

6-oz (full fat) Greek yogurt
1-tbsp organic honey
1-tbsp crushed walnuts or almonds
½-cup berries

Add yogurt to a small serving bowl. Drizzle with honey and sprinkle with nuts and berries. Serves 1.

Scrambled Eggs with Mushrooms and Turkey

2 large eggs
1/8-tsp salt
1/8-tsp pepper
1-tbsp olive oil
3-oz shredded turkey
2 thinly sliced mushrooms

Add olive oil to a pre-heated skillet. Stir-fry turkey and mushrooms until mushrooms are soft. Whisk both eggs and add salt and pepper. Add egg mixture to skillet and stir slowly. Cook until done to personal preference. Slide onto a small plate and serves 1.

Lunch Recipes

You want lunch to be food that brings you high energy and lasting power. Both of these give you a savory flavor experience and tantalizing combinations of textures. One powers you with antioxidant-rich sweet potatoes and healthy fat chicken. The other uses the power of low-carb veggies and protein-rich nuts and egg, mellowed with high-healthy fat avocado. Both are wise combinations that blend and balance the needs of your body at this important high-energy time of the day.

Sweet Potatoes with Cream and Chicken

1-6 oz chicken breast
1-large sweet potato cubed
½-cup sliced onion
1-minced garlic clove
½-cup heavy cream
1-tsp salt
1-tsp pepper
3-cups water

Add all ingredients to slow cooker. Set on low and let cook for 6 to 8 hours. Serves 1.

Late-Summer Salad with Figs

Salad:
2-handfuls spinach leaves
3-4 quartered fresh figs
3-4 sliced cherry tomatoes
½ large avocado, pitted, peeled, and sliced
8-10 almonds or cashews

1-large, soft-boiled egg, halved

Dressing:
1/4 cup apple cider vinegar
½ lemon squeezed
½-tsp sea salt
½-tsp pepper
1-tbsp olive oil

Layer a plate with spinach leaves. Add a layer of avocado. Evenly distribute the tomatoes, figs, and nuts. Place the egg on top, center of dish. Sprinkle liberally with mixed dressing. Serves 1.

Dinner Recipes

What do both of these dinners have in common? The greens and vegetables paired with a nice healthy fat meat. High protein, moderate carbs, and high healthy fat. The perfect dinner combination. Filling and delicious.

Quinoa Salad with Salmon and Corn

½-cup dry quinoa
1 ½-cups chicken or vegetable stock
Salt to taste
Pepper to taste
1-tbsp olive oil
2-fillet of salmon, skin on, about 1-inch thick,
4-oz each
2-cups loosely packed baby spinach
½-cup corn
2-tbsp fresh basil, roughly chopped
¼-tsp cumin

Add quinoa and stock to a small pot and bring
to a boil. Stir and cook for 15 minutes. Set it
covered away from the heat for 5 minutes.
Fluff with a fork and set aside.

Add ½ of the olive oil to a skillet over medium
heat. Place salmon in with skin-side down.
Cook for 4 minutes and flip. Lower heat
slightly and cook 2 minutes. Flip again and
cook 2 more minutes.

Mix the spinach, corn, remaining olive oil,
basil, quinoa, and cumin together. Place on

two plates and cover each with a salmon fillet. Sprinkle with salt and pepper to taste. Serves 2.

Grilled Steak with Roasted Potatoes

2-lbs skirt or flank steak
½-cup olive oil
7-cloves garlic, 4 crushed, 3 sliced
5-sprigs of fresh parsley
5-7 small red potatoes, quartered
Salt to taste
Pepper to taste
2-cups fresh green beans

Add 6-tbsp olive oil, garlic, steak, and parsley in a resealable bag. Rub ingredients on the steak and set aside to marinate for an hour.

Toss crushed garlic, olive oil, and potatoes in a bowl and place onto baking sheet. Sprinkle with salt and pepper. Place in a 450-degree oven for 20 minutes. Turn every few minutes.

Add green beans to a small pot of boiling water and let simmer for 15 minutes, drain and set aside.

Brush skillet with olive oil and heat over medium heat. Add steaks and let cook for 7 minutes each side for medium-rare results. Let meat rest for 5 minutes. Slice thin and serve with potatoes and green beans. Serves 2.

Dessert Recipes

Treats like this are not going to be on your list for every evening but it makes a nice sweet treat occasionally. They do tend to be somewhat high in sugars and carbs. It's okay to enjoy a little indulgence now and again. It's also packed with plenty of healthy fats and antioxidant-rich fruit. You can trade nearly any fruit in both recipes.

Caramelized Pears

½-stick unsalted butter
½-cup light packed brown sugar
4-medium pears, pitted and cubed
¼-tsp ground allspice

Melt butter in a skillet over medium heat. Add brown sugar once butter is completely melted. Stir well. Add pear cubes and allspice. Allow the pears to sit in the pan with sugar, spice, and butter mixture for a couple of minutes between stirs. Remove from heat once it has caramelized. Place a heaping serving spoon in each bowl. Serves 2-3.

Frozen Raspberry Pie

Crust:
12-14 whole graham crackers
6-tbsp butter, melted

Pie filling:
2 cups heavy cream
¾-cup sugar
4-cups raspberries
1-tbsp fresh lemon juice

Create pie crust by pulsing graham crackers in a blender until crumb texture, mix into melted butter and press into the bottom of a 9-inch pie pan (freezer safe).

Make pie filling by adding the heavy cream and 2-tbsp sugar to a mixing bowl. Use a mixer and beat until it begins to form peaks. Add raspberries, the remainder of sugar and lemon juice to the blender. Puree and separate seeds from the liquid. Add liquid to the heavy cream/sugar mixture until well blended. Place in the pie crust and freeze for 8 hours or overnight. Slice and serve. 14 servings.

Conclusion

Thank you for making it through to the end of *Intermittent Fasting for Women*. Let's hope it was informative and able to provide you with all of the tools you need to achieve your goals whatever they may be.

You now have one of the best sources of information and instruction on IF plans for women that are available on the market. Now it's time for you to begin your journaling and prepare to make the changes necessary to give you the results you want. IF is less about a diet and more about a complete lifestyle change. A change that focuses on your health and well-being. It's time to quit putting yourself last!

IF isn't a crazy fad diet that promises things too impossible to achieve. It uses a real, all-natural process within your own body to initiate and accelerate fat burning without the use of harmful chemicals and diet pills. As long as you are in reasonable health, it can be done safely with very little side effect or complication.

Turn back the clock on your body at the deepest cellular levels with the detox power that only fasting can provide. Feel healthier, invigorated, with energy levels you haven't had in years! Find the IF plan you like or switch it up every now and again to keep it interesting. You have complete control over the level of fasting and fat burning you want to achieve.

Combine forces with the IF plan of your choice and a ketogenic diet to get consistent weight loss and tons of other health benefits. The ketogenic diet and fasting help your body heal and repair from the inside out. Every cell in your body will feel the rejuvenation from day one. Say goodbye to the cellular clutter that leads to illness and even cancer.

Every woman at every stage of life can benefit from Intermittent Fasting. You can finally enjoy more stable weight management with a safe increase in metabolism. It will completely change your relationship with food.

Finally, if you found this book useful in any way, a review on Amazon is always appreciated!